Thyroid Problems

IN WOMEN
AND CHILDREN

Self-Help and Treatment

Joan Gomez, M.D.

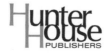

Hunter House Inc., Publishers
PO Box 2914
Alameda CA 94501-0914

Library of Congress Cataloging-in-Publication Data

Gomez, Joan.
Thyroid problems in women and children : self-help and treatment / Joan Gomez.
    p. cm.
Includes bibliographical references and index.
    ISBN 0-89793-385-0 (pbk. : alk. paper) — ISBN 0-89793-386-9 (cloth : alk. paper)
1. Thyroid gland—Diseases. 2. Thyroid gland diseases in pregnancy. 3. Women—Diseases. 4. Children—Diseases. I. Title.
RC655 .G667 2003
616.4'4—dc21   2002151931

Project Credits

Cover Design: Brian Dittmar Graphic
    Design
Book Production: Jil Weil/Hunter House
Developmental and Copy Editor:
    Kelley Blewster
Proofreader: John David Marion
Indexer: Nancy D. Peterson
Acquisitions Editor: Jeanne Brondino
Editor: Alexandra Mummery
Editorial Assistant: Caroline Knapp

Sales and Marketing Coordinator:
    Jo Anne Retzlaff
Publicity Coordinator:
    Earlita K. Chenault
Customer Service Manager:
    Christina Sverdrup
Order Fulfillment: Lakdhon Lama
Administrator: Theresa Nelson
Computer Support: Peter Eichelberger
Publisher: Kiran S. Rana

Printed and Bound by Transcontinental Printing, Canada

9 8 7 6 5 4 3 2 1   First Edition   03 04 05 06 07

Contents

IMPORTANT NOTE

The material in this book is intended to provide a review of resources and information related to thyroid problems. Every effort has been made to provide accurate and dependable information. However, professionals in the field may have differing opinions, and change is always taking place. Any of the treatments described herein should be undertaken only under the guidance of a licensed health-care practitioner. The author, editors, and publishers cannot be held responsible for any error, omission, professional disagreement, outdated material, or adverse outcomes that derive from use of any of these treatments or information resources in this book, either in a program of self-care or under the care of a licensed practitioner.

Introduction

I empathize with people who have thyroid problems because they have cropped up in my family, too. The very first thing I did when I became a doctor was to take my mother to see a thyroid specialist. My mother had an unsightly bulge in the front of her neck—easily cured, although she'd had it for as long as I could remember. Much later my daughter, a brilliant student, started slowing down and not coping well. By that time I had developed an interest in the thyroid, and we were able to nip the problem in the bud.

Thyroid disease affects an estimated thirteen to fourteen million Americans, and as many as one-half to two-thirds of those affected don't even know they have the problem. Depending on the specific thyroid condition, five to ten times as many women as men suffer from thyroid disorders. (See the end of Chapter 1 for more about the prevalence of thyroid disorders in the United States.) Thyroid illness in American children is fairly rare (only about one in four thousand are born with thyroid underactivity, for example). However, thyroid problems that occur in newborns are critical and must be addressed within a few months of birth; if they are not, mental retardation or even death can be the dire consequences. Thyroid problems that occur in older children can easily go unnoticed; awareness and education on the parents' part is crucial for detecting them.

That's where this book can help. *Thyroid Problems in Women and Children: Self-Help and Treatment* outlines in detail the warning signs of thyroid disease in women and youngsters of all ages and offers suggestions for what to do when one or more of those signs is detected. Fortunately, treatment of most thyroid illnesses, in both adults and children, is relatively simple and enjoys a high success rate, as you will also learn from reading this book.

It may have been quite a shock to you when your doctor suggested doing thyroid tests. Perhaps you had gone to see him hoping he would prescribe something to buck you up because you were feeling so down—tired, sluggish, cold all the time, and, to add to your discomfort, constipated. Everything seemed to take twice as long and require twice the effort, and all this had crept up on you so sneakily. These symptoms are unpleasant, to be sure, but if the test results came back as "underactive thyroid," take heart—you are actually in luck. An underactive thyroid is a common disorder. It can affect you at any age, but it is rather more likely to occur as you get older. The treatment consists of taking tiny white tablets to supplement your own supply of thyroid hormones. They work like magic, and they have no side effects. You will feel yourself gradually coming back to life again—and shedding those few unwanted pounds in the process.

On the other hand, you may have gone to the doctor wanting help with something quite different—your nerves. You may have started feeling anxious all the time, for no reason. You couldn't sit still, you'd fly off the handle at the slightest thing, and your heart kept thumping. Although your appetite was enormous, you were losing weight, and that was a worry. These are the signs of an overactive thyroid. Sometimes the symptoms seem to come on after a shock, but usually no one knows why, out of the blue, the thyroid gland has started overworking. Fortunately, there is a range of medicines that will calm it down, and your mind and your heart will follow suit. Your body will run at its normal, peaceful pace again.

Or perhaps you've noticed a prominent bulge in the front of your neck, indicating a swelling of the thyroid gland. This condition is unimportant in itself from the health point of view. In some cases, for instance during pregnancy, it can be normal and temporary. In others it is due to either an overactive or an underactive thyroid, and shrinks down as the problem is settled.

It may, however, be your child you are worried about—he or she isn't growing as quickly as other children, or is shooting up faster than they are. Either way, he or she is not doing well in school. Again, the remedy is straightforward.

As noted, thyroid problems affect women significantly more often than men or children, and my impression is that those affected are usually particularly warm, sympathetic people. Sometimes a thyroid malfuntion comes to light from some apparently unrelated symptom, such as heavy, irregular menstrual periods, or a near cessation of menstruation; fertility difficulties; problems in swallowing; or, in some older people, high blood pressure and certain heart conditions. These conditions, too, all respond to treatment that returns the thyroid to good working order.

What does it mean once a thyroid disorder has been diagnosed? Particularly if your thyroid is overactive, when the disorder itself makes you nervous, you may be worried about what the treatment entails. Nearly always, it only amounts to swallowing tablets. Sometimes this is for a short course, but in the case of an underactive thyroid it may be indefinitely. None of the treatments work immediately, but after two weeks, as a rule, you should experience an end to the worst discomfort. After that it is mainly a matter of fine-tuning the dosage. With an overactive thyroid, different medicines may be needed at different stages of recovery.

You may have heard of radioactive iodine as a treatment for an overactive thyroid. It sounds quite frightening, but it has been used for many years and is so safe that it is now recommended even for children. All that is needed for a permanent cure is to take radioactive iodine (in tablet or liquid form) once, and then wait. The treatment introduces very little radioactivity to the body as a whole, but a great deal to the thyroid. The radioactivity lasts only a few hours, but the beneficial effect comes on gradually, over several months.

As was the case in my family, thyroid problems, but not necessarily the same kind, often run in families. This is because they are mostly caused by autoimmunity—the body's making a mistake and reacting against itself. Since thyroid disorders are 90 percent curable, don't worry if they crop up among your relatives. If they do, and if you're diligent about providing your doctor with a good family medical history, then he or she will be alert to thyroid problems in you, even if all you exhibit are the less straightforward symptoms.

While you are preoccupied with digesting the news of a thyroid disorder, you won't be able to take in every word your doctor says, especially if she slips into using medical jargon. In *Thyroid Problems in Women and Children* I aim to share with you all the information you are ever likely to need about the thyroid, in understandable language and right up-to-date. After the opening chapter explains the physiological importance of your thyroid, the following three chapters are each devoted to a common thyroid disorder (enlarged thyroid, underactive thyroid, and overactive thyroid). Next, several chapters address thyroid problems in some of the critical life stages in women and children (pregnancy and birth, infancy, childhood and adolescence, and the senior years). Chapter 9 focuses on issues related to calcitonin—the "other" thyroid hormone.

The book's final two chapters—on keeping your thyroid happy and on common thyroid tests and treatments—can be viewed as overviews or digests of information that in some cases is also discussed in earlier chapters. The difference is that in these two chapters the information is located all together in one place and is organized in convenient reference format.

I hope reading this book gives you the confidence to ask questions and get the best out of your discussions with your doctor. Most of all, I hope it helps you to avoid the sort of worrying that comes from not knowing what the disorder and its treatment involve.

Postscript: My mother had no further trouble with her thyroid and lived until she was ninety-five, and my daughter has enjoyed sparkling health for years.

What Your Thyroid Does for You

What is so special about your thyroid? In fact, it could not have a more important role. It is in charge of running every part of your body, including how you feel emotionally. As you can imagine, if it goes wrong you are affected all over, whatever your age, sex, or race. Yet it is a seemingly insignificant slip of tissue, weighing about an ounce (30 grams). It fits so neatly into the space around the lower part of your voice box—your larynx—that you wouldn't know it was there unless you knew how to find it.

To locate your thyroid, look in a mirror and swallow. You will see your larynx move up and down at the front of your neck. Lean your head forward and feel each side of your larynx with your fingers and thumb. You can just detect a little bit of soft tissue closely attached to the sides of the larynx, making them feel less hard than the front part. This is your thyroid. Its name dates from the seventeenth century and comes from the Greek word for *shield*—after the shape of a Minoan battle shield.

The thyroid controls the body by producing hormones. The word *hormone* comes from the Greek word for *stimulator*, which is exactly what the thyroid hormones are. These chemical messengers boost activity all over the body. They travel in the bloodstream. Since every single part of the body must have its nourishment supplied through the blood for survival, it follows that hormones are also conveyed to every body part. The thyroid is small, but it is so busy and important that it has a wonderfully generous blood supply. Five times its own weight of blood goes through the gland every minute.

Not every organ or tissue needs a particular hormone in the same amount all the time, so a system is in place that is rather like leaving a note out for the milkman. The parts that require more hormones open up more receptors, which latch on to the hormones. Fewer receptors are opened up when less hormone is required. Thus, the right quantity is supplied to the right place at the right time.

The next several sections describe the various mechanisms through which the thyroid and its hormones influence your health and everyday functioning.

METABOLISM

The essential work of the body is called *metabolism*, from the Greek word for *change*. Metabolism involves taking in adequate amounts of food and processing it to provide energy to keep the heart, breathing, and digestion going; to fuel the muscles as and when needed; and to keep the brain running. It involves repair and replacement of tissues on a regular schedule, and the disposal of waste. Another metabolic task is the conversion of alcohol and medicines into a form in which the body can get rid of them. Imagine the chaos that would ensue if every cocktail or every aspirin you swallowed remained unprocessed in your body.

One of the thyroid's most important jobs is to monitor and control your metabolic rate—the rate at which your body uses its fuel reserves. If there are heavy calls on your fuel reserves from your muscles because you are playing tennis or doing a spring cleaning, or from your digestive system because there is a big meal waiting to be dealt with, your metabolic rate accel-

erates. The orders for an increase in metabolism com
thyroid.

Incidentally, a meal that is high in protein is hard work to
digest; it therefore stimulates the metabolic reaction much more
than a fatty meal. That is why weight-loss diets used to feature
steak prominently, in the hope of inducing the metabolism to
burn away unwanted flesh faster. The Russian diet, except for
that eaten by the wealthy, contains a lot of oil and hardly any
meat. This encourages the bulky figures we used to see in Red
Square on television.

Several factors affect the metabolic rate; the remainder of
this section describes some of them.

Basal Metabolic Rate

If you are doing nothing more energetic than, say, reading this
book, your bodily functions will be just ticking along. In such
circumstances, your metabolic rate will sink to its basic minimum—the basal metabolic rate, or BMR—under the guidance of
the thyroid. The BMR remains high throughout childhood,
when the body is undergoing active growth and making new tissues, and in pregnancy, another building period. It also stays high
during breast-feeding. Thyroid hormone is particularly involved
in the manufacture of body protein, especially muscle tissue,
either your own or an unborn baby's, or for milk production.
The BMR settles down in ordinary adult life and middle age, but
it decreases once you enter the contemplative phase of old age.

Geographical Climate

If you move to a colder climate, your BMR will rev up by as
much as 50 percent after a few weeks, again under the direction
of the thyroid. This happens because you have to burn bodily
fuel faster to produce more warmth. Such vital internal organs
as the liver and kidneys cannot work properly unless they maintain a normal temperature, regardless of the temperature of the
hands and feet. People who live in the Arctic regions run at a

consistently higher BMR, by 15 to 20 percent, than those of us in, say, London or New York. A small adjustment in the metabolic rate occurs between winter and summer even in temperate climates, and you will notice the instinct to take in bigger supplies of food in a cold snap. (A special tissue called *brown fat* is especially useful for producing heat. It is concentrated along the back. Babies, and to a lesser extent young men, have plenty of this material. The fat of the middle-aged has no such useful, warming function, but remains inert, padding the figure.)

If you live at or travel to high altitudes, the thyroid increases metabolic activity due to the reduced concentration of oxygen in the atmosphere. Serious mountaineers must acclimatize themselves before tackling the highest peaks. Exposure to long sunlit days also stimulates extra thyroid-hormone production and increased metabolism, although hot weather has the opposite effect.

Eating and Appetite

Another useful maneuver of the thyroid is the adjustment of both basic and short-term rates of metabolism in response to how much a person eats, though it doesn't respond to actual body weight. If you persistently take in more food than your body needs, the thyroid will help to dispose of the surplus by having it burn up more rapidly. This automatically makes you feel warmer, whatever the temperature. You can see this mechanism in action next time you go to a restaurant. You are sure to spot one or two hearty eaters looking hot and flushed; they are burning fuel fast.

By contrast, if you are on short rations—whether by choice because you are dieting or because the food is unavailable—your thyroid will eke out the body's needed sustenance from the available food supply by slowing down the metabolism. This is what happens in anorexia nervosa. A low metabolic rate makes a person feel deadly cold, and if it continues for long her health suffers.

Appetite is influenced by the thyroid, which nudges it toward what the body really needs. Since you are a free agent, you can, of course, override this sensible guidance. If you have been off your food because of a cold or an upset stomach, as you recover you find yourself craving simple, easy-to-digest, nourishing foods until you are back to normal. Often the thyroid dampens the appetite during the working week to compensate for a little indulgence on the weekend.

Unfortunately, the influence of the thyroid on appetite and metabolic rate depends not on how fat or thin you are, but on whether you are taking in more—or less—than you can use, particularly in comparison with what you have previously eaten. An overweight person who is trying to lose weight by eating very little will have a slow metabolic rate, so that he or she is burning the food reserves only very slowly—the reverse of what is wanted. At the same time, to make matters worse, the appetite will be pressing for more!

You may have noticed that men in general have bigger appetites than women. This is because they have a higher BMR. Young men and small babies have brown fat, which produces more energy than any other tissue and lights up like a lamp in response to excess food or cold. Men also have a brisker burning-off reaction than women if they overeat or when they exercise.

Another way the thyroid helps the body is by turning down the metabolism and reducing appetite during certain illnesses. This releases the body from the tasks of digestion, so that all its energies can go toward repair and recovery.

LOOKS

Not only are a person's metabolism and weight affected by the thyroid, it also has some influence on one's general appearance: the glossiness and luxuriousness, or otherwise, of one's hair; whether the skin is thick or delicate, dry or moist; and to some extent the shape of the face and hands. More important with regard to how other people see you is your vitality—the physical and mental energy that shines through all you do. The thyroid plays a role in both aspects, appearance and vitality.

OTHER BODILY FUNCTIONS

The thyroid acts as a long-term pacemaker for heartbeat, breathing, and other regular bodily functions such as bowel action and menstrual periods. The timing of these may all be modified by circumstances—that is, the heart rate speeds up with excitement or physical exertion, the bowels move faster on a high-fiber diet—but the underlying rates and rhythms are set by the thyroid. The action of the thyroid also causes your heart rate and breathing to soon settle back to "normal" (whatever that means for you in particular) when you sit down after running for a bus, for example.

Muscular efficiency, for sports or work, depends on the right amount of thyroid hormone: too little and your muscles are stiff and slow to move; too much and you feel exhausted after achieving very little. Various rheumatic and joint problems are associated with thyroid disorder.

Nowadays we are constantly warned about the dangers of too high a level of cholesterol in the blood. It increases the risks of heart attack and stroke, especially for men. One of the tasks of thyroid hormone is to keep the cholesterol level in check—but this is a vain attempt in the seriously overweight.

MENTAL AND EMOTIONAL BALANCE

Health is usually considered from the physical aspect, but you are more than just a body. The essential you lies in your mind and personality. Your confidence and drive, your mental energy, depends on an adequate supply of thyroid hormone. If thyroid-hormone levels are normal, you will be alert but not on edge, and your concentration will be sharp and focused. You will be able to express yourself without difficulty and solve day-to-day problems, in the absence of illness or a major disaster.

More importantly for a happy life, if your thyroid is in balance, so too will be your judgement. You will neither panic over trivia nor sink into helpless despair at the first setback. You will steer between unrealistic optimism and the propensity to see only the black side. Sexual feeling—libido—and ordinary friendliness also both depend in part on the thyroid.

BIOLOGICAL TIMEKEEPING

A properly working thyroid is of crucial importance during the developmental stages. It is the thyroid that "tells" each body part at the appropriate time when and how to grow, in accordance with the genetic blueprint provided by the parents. The unborn baby's thyroid goes into hormone production from about the third month of gestation, but the baby still requires a supply of the hormone from his or her mother.

Birth is a dramatic event from any viewpoint, including that of the thyroid. As soon as the umbilical cord is cut, the baby's thyroid springs into action, flooding the bloodstream with hormones. This very high level reaches a peak about the second day after birth, and continues for six to eight weeks. Growth and development run the metabolism at its maximum. It is because of the high metabolic rate induced by the thyroid, and the presence of brown fat, that tiny babies survive under circumstances that would cause adults to perish. Babies buried under rubble in the 1985 Mexican earthquake lived without warmth or nourishment for days after rescuers were abandoning hope of finding anyone alive. Premature babies, however, lack this remarkable thyroid reaction to coming into the cold world. They must live in an incubator until their thyroid is sufficiently mature.

Throughout childhood the thyroid plays an important role in growth and development, particularly of the bones and teeth, and of the brain and nervous system. A child's height and the timing of her or his first and second sets of teeth are of interest, but not of such vital importance as mental and emotional development. For children, this includes behavior, bathroom training, and how they do in school, both intellectually and socially. An underactive thyroid is far more damaging than an overactive one. To anticipate any of these problems, today all babies born in the West have their thyroid function checked at birth.

Problems arising later are less serious, and once recognized can be treated effectively. At puberty, the thyroid is again actively involved in the changes that occur in turning a child into a man or woman. If a human adolescent is short of thyroid hormone, at seventeen he or she will look like a ten-year-old—short and childlike, with underdeveloped sexual organs. The secondary characteristics will be delayed, too—breast development and menstruation for girls, change of voice and facial hair for boys.

WOMEN AND THE THYROID

The creation of the next generation depends on healthy thyroid glands in today's adults, especially the females. If the thyroid is either overactive or underactive, fertility plummets in either sex. In general, however, thyroid problems affect women much more often than men because estrogen, the female sex hormone, makes women more responsive to the fluctuating effects of thyroid hormone than men. Alternatively, men's sex hormones— the androgens—have the opposite effect.

The ever-running female cycle of preparation in case of conception, followed by the menstrual period; the miracle of pregnancy and later of making milk; and the dramatic sign-off at menopause are essential female concerns. Each of these female conditions requires the correct thyroid input.

A woman's emotional system is also more susceptible to upset than a man's. Even minor thyroid disorders can bring on depression or a state of anxiety in a woman, while men are affected only by serious thyroid dysfunction. There are two stages in a woman's life when she is particularly vulnerable to fluctuations in thyroid-hormone levels, and especially to their effect on emotions: after giving birth and at menopause. At each of these times a sharp falloff occurs in the production of the female sex hormone, because of reduced need. At the same time, a small reduction takes place in the need for thyroid hormone. If thyroid-hormone production temporarily drops off too much, a new mother may be depressed and low in energy. The same is true with a menopausal woman. By contrast, if the thyroid keeps operating normally, without much of a dip in its output of hormone, the mother will be less likely to experience postpartum depression, and the fifty-year-old less likely to endure the discomforts of hot flashes, low moods, and weight gain. (However, it should be noted that probably more women blame their thyroid for middle-age spread than is truly justified.)

OTHER STRESSES

The thyroid interacts with the two stress hormones: cortisol, the body's own steroid, and adrenaline, the emergency hormone. Thyroid activity goes down when cortisol is called into play, but it enhances the action of adrenaline. Thyroid hormone is also increased in repsonse to the stress of taking an exam or during a surgical operation; this occurs because the metabolism of most tissues (except in the brain) is increased at such times.

WHAT ARE THE THYROID HORMONES?

The thyroid hormones are the only hormones that contain iodine as a key ingredient. The gland takes the iodine it needs from the circulating blood and within minutes converts it into a form in which it can be stored for use as and when needed.

A normal diet contains more than enough iodine to supply the thyroid. All it needs is about one milligram (mg) a week—a quantity too small to see. Iodine is present in various foods, tap water, and milk. In some inland and mountainous areas there is a shortage of iodine in the soil, which can cause problems if the inhabitants produce all their food locally. This doesn't apply in

Western and other developed countries, since our food comes from many sources. Iodized salt is no longer considered necessary anywhere in the United Kingdom, though it is still available in the United States.

Too much iodine is as bad as too little. As with some vitamins and other minerals, an excess is toxic and particularly upsets the thyroid. It is unwise to take any extra iodine unless your doctor specifically advises it.

The two major thyroid hormones are referred to as T_4 (thyroxine) and T_3 (triiodothyronine). Each chemical unit, or molecule, of T_4 contains four atoms of iodine; each molecule of T_3 has three. Ninety percent of the thyroid output is T_4; 10 percent is T_3. They both have the same stimulating effect, but T_3 is four times as powerful as T_4 and works eight times as fast.

A neat arrangement allows T_4 to turn into T_3 at the drop of a hat by shedding one of its iodine atoms. This happens onsite—that is, in the body part, for example the leg muscles, where an immediate boost to the metabolism is required. On the other hand, there may be a call to reduce the metabolic rate—because of low fuel reserves due to dieting, or an illness that requires minimal use of the body's resources. In this situation there is an efficient shutdown of the slow T_4 and fast T_3 stimulating effects, by the conversion of T_4 into so-called reverse-T_3, which does not stimulate the metabolism.

The thyroid keeps a store of iodine (attached to big protein molecules), and up to three months' reserve of almost-ready-to-use T_4—sort of like those prepared meals you can buy at the supermarket that just need heating up when you want them.

HOW DOES THE THYROID KNOW HOW MUCH HORMONE TO MAKE?

Like all the other hormone producers—the ovaries, testes, adrenals, pancreas, placenta, and embyro—the thyroid comes under direct orders from the great coordinator, the pituitary. The pituitary transmits instructions by special, individual hormones; in the case of the thyroid, it releases thyroid-stimulating hormone, or TSH, when it wants to instruct the gland to produce and/or secrete more hormone.

The pituitary comes under the direction of the highest authority of all: the hypothalamus, in conjunction with the limbic system, which is wrapped around it and which affects both the emotions and the automatic control of body functions. The hypothalamus is a sliver of brain tissue located in the safest possible place, the center of the head. It is your personal communications center, continuously monitoring information from all parts of the body, for instance a fall in blood-sugar levels or an itch in the right big toe. It collects and analyzes the incoming information and sets off various reactions. Its purpose is to keep everything running steadily, for instance your bodily temperature, modifying it by causing sweating or shivering if necessary; water balance; sleep-waking cycle; menstrual cycle; blood chemistry; sexual activity; etc.

In addition to the input of practical information, every nuance of feeling—pleasure, guilt, fear, or contentment—every hope and desire, short- or long-term, and also your (free) will is conveyed to the hypothalamus. It collates all this information—practical, imaginative, and feeling—and programs the pituitary by a superfast hotline. The pituitary, tucked under the brain, then instructs the body's numerous departments and coordinates them all, like the conductor of a magical orchestra. Modern microchip technology is nothing compared with the marvellous subtlety of the hormonal apparatus we all have.

ONE MORE HORMONE

It was not until the 1970s that another hormone, totally unlike T_3 and T_4, was discovered in the thyroid. Its name is *calcitonin*, because it helps to control the amount of calcium in the blood and bones. It is given as a medicine in the treatment of Paget's disease, a problem affecting some elderly people in which certain bones become enlarged. A blood test for calcitonin has also proved useful in providing an early warning for medullary thyroid cancer and oat-cell cancers of the lung, breast, and pancreas.

THYROID DISEASE IN THE UNITED STATES

As you can imagine after reading about the thyroid gland's involvement in so many vital bodily processes, thyroid problems can cause you to feel bad—or, even worse, can seriously affect your health—in many different ways. The dangers of having an untreated thyroid disease include a greater risk of osteoporosis, heart and artery disorders, problems in the nervous system, and an excess of cholesterol in the blood—all potential killers. For this reason thyroid disease is a significant public-health concern.

Just how common are thyroid disorders? Unlike with most illnesses, thyroid disease is quite a bit less prevalent in the United States than it is in Europe. However, three new studies, published in the *Journal of Clinical Endocrinology and Metabolism* in 2002, trumpet the widespread prevalence of thyroid disease in the United States and its significant effects. Researchers at the Centers for Disease Control and Prevention (CDC) checked out seventeen thousand people with the two standard blood tests for thyroid malfunction: TSH and T_4, plus another for thyroid antibodies. The subjects tested were drawn from the National Health and Nutrition Survey of the U.S. population between 1988 and 1994. They were all over twelve years old and represented the same geographical and ethnic characteristics as the population in general.

The researchers found that 5 percent of Americans had thyroid disorders of which they were unaware; four-fifths of these showed the signs of underactive thyroid. Proportionately more white and Mexican Americans than blacks were affected. Women and older people also figured largely among those with diagnosable thyroid disease.

Dr. Joseph Hollowell, the leader of the CDC study, recommends more screening, especially for those at particular risk—for instance those with a family history of thyroid problems or autoimmune disorders. Middle-aged and older women are the most vulnerable. The sooner the diagnosis of a thyroid abnormality is made and treatment started, the better the chances of sidestepping the complications.

So what exactly are these serious-sounding conditions, such as "underactive thyroid" and "autoimmune disorders," and how might they affect you? Keep reading. More about all of these topics is provided in the rest of the book. Armed with this information, you will be well equipped to understand any thyroid problem you or a family member is diagnosed with, to work with your health-care providers in implementing the appropriate preventive and therapeutic measures—and to enhance your thyroid health.

2

Enlarged Thyroid

Swelling of the neck from an oversize thyroid has been recognized since history was first recorded. The condition has had a variety of names, including struma, botium, galagande, gongrona, choiron, and the one that has stuck: goiter. For centuries it was considered an enhancement of beauty, probably because it so often occurred in girls in their teens and twenties. Cleopatra is depicted with a goiter in a relief at Dendera, in the Nile Valley, and Rubens's charming painting of his sister-in-law (*Le Chapeau de Paille*, hanging in the National Gallery, London) shows a pretty, sprightly young woman with a big hat and a noticeably large thyroid.

Like everything to do with the thyroid, goiter affects more women than men, but not exclusively. Around 1550, Michelangelo's surgeon pointed out for the first time that females in general have larger thyroid glands than men, although Michelangelo himself developed a big thyroid. In the margin of a sonnet he wrote for a friend, he drew a sketch of himself with the typical bulge at the front of his neck, and annotated it, "I've grown a goiter by dwelling in this den." The "den" was the Sistine Chapel, which was taking him a long time to paint.

There are seven principal types of thyroid enlargement, which we will look at in turn:

1. normal, physiological goiter

2. simple goiter

3. multinodular goiter

4. nodular goiter

5. endemic goiter (from iodine deficiency or other chemical effects)

6. autoimmune goiter (several types)

7. thyroid tumor (benign or cancerous)

NORMAL, PHYSIOLOGICAL GOITER

During Adolescence

Throughout childhood there is no difference in appearance between boys' and girls' necks. That changes at puberty. When boys' voices are breaking and their larynx—or Adam's apple—is becoming more prominent, girls of the same age tend to have a smoother, fuller look at the front of the neck, and it is quite common for there to be an actual bulge, or goiter. Most likely a friend or the doctor will be the first to notice it. Since there is neither discomfort nor tenderness and the youngster is perfectly fit, there is nothing to draw her attention to it.

The explanation lies in the teenage surge of sex hormones circulating through the body, particularly estrogen in the case of a girl, in response to the maturation of the ovaries. Estrogen in turn has a stimulating effect on the thyroid. The thyroid responds by working harder to meet the increased need for hormones, and like a muscle after exercise, it increases in size to an extent that may be noticeable. The gland does not produce more than is needed of its own hormones, so there are no general effects on the body. None of this happens in boys, because male sex hormones—androgens—tend to have a dampening effect on the thyroid.

Annabel was getting ready for her sixteenth-birthday party. As she clipped on the gold necklace she had been given the previous year, she was surprised to find it slightly tight. Looking at her neck in the mirror, she could see a distinct bulge that hadn't been there earlier. Then she remembered Aunt May, who had to have an operation for her thyroid. Annabel was scared and arranged to see her doctor. She was told not to worry, that in her case it was just a part of normal growing up. She was to come back in six months for a check. Putting on the same necklace for her eighteenth-birthday celebration, Annabel found it was now comfortably loose again.

During Pregnancy

Even more than during adolescence, in pregnancy there is an increased supply of estrogen, and a need for greater thyroid activity to provide for the growing fetus. The gland often becomes measurably bigger. The Roman poet Catullus, in about 50 B.C., described a state-of-the-art pregnancy test. A thread was tied around the woman's throat; if it became tight or broke, that was positive. The term *honeymoon goiter* referred to the probability of pregnancy in the days before reliable contraception.

Other sources of extra estrogen may mimic pregnancy and deceive the thyroid into doing extra work. They include the contraceptive pill and HRT (hormone replacement therapy). These may stimulate swelling of the thyroid. Cannabis acts similarly if used regularly.

Physiological enlargement of the thyroid does not usually persist after the rhythm of the periods is well established in an adolescent, or after about six to eight weeks following pregnancy. Sometimes, however, instead of reverting to its previous, undetectable state, the thyroid remains big and may gradually get bigger. This is one type of simple goiter.

SIMPLE GOITER

Simple goiter is enlargement of a healthy thyroid gland, but accompanied by neither overproduction nor underproduction of thyroid hormones. The commonest form of simple goiter world-wide is the endemic type (see below). Aside from the endemic type, it has been estimated that around 5 percent of people in the United States develop a simple goiter at some time in their lives. This may simply be a continuation of the physiological swelling of puberty or pregnancy, but it can also crop up out of the blue, affecting some men as well as women. The gland commonly enlarges to two or three times its normal size—which is still not very noticeable—though it may become huge.

The enlarged thyroid is smooth, symmetrical, and soft to the touch. The likeliest age for it to appear is between fifteen and twenty-five, and there is a good chance of its returning to its earlier size over two or three years. It is unlikely to cause any problems, except possibly a slight feeling of tightness at times when swallowing.

What to Do

The first step is to have a discussion with your doctor, so that he or she is aware of the situation. Unless he or she finds something else when examining you, treatment is unnecessary from the point of view of your health. If the bulge annoys you by its presence, the doctor may think it worthwhile to give you a small daily dose of thyroxine (thyroid hormone) to encourage the gland to shrink. This seems to help in some cases, but not all. In the uncommon event that the goiter becomes unsightly or uncomfortable due to its size, you may decide to have a tidying-up operation. This is more often required by older people with the multinodular type of goiter (see below).

MULTINODULAR GOITER

In multinodular goiter, instead of being smooth like a cushion, the gland develops an irregular, lumpy consistency. The change may be noticeable to the feel, and it may involve more or less enlargement. Multinodular goiter may develop over ten or twenty years from a simple, smooth swelling that never goes away, but it can also crop up out of nowhere, and, unlike simple goiter, it stays. The peak age range when it appears is between thirty-five and fifty-five. A mild degree of the condition is extremely common, probably affecting 60 percent of middle-aged women, many of them unaware of it.

The thyroid is still producing the appropriate quota of hormones, so there are no general symptoms. From around age sixty onward there is a slightly greater likelihood of the condition's causing local pressure problems. Pressure on the windpipe—called *tracheal compression*—can make breathing noisy at times, while slight pressure on the gullet can cause discomfort when swallowing a hard chunk of meat, for instance.

NODULAR GOITER

This is the term used to indicate a single noticeable lump or nodule in or on the thyroid, which is otherwise working normally. Usually other nodular parts are also present that aren't visible.

Up to 50 percent of the U.S. population will develop a lump or nodule on their thyroid at some time in their lives. These are usually harmless, but so-called "hot" nodules produce an excess of thyroid hormone, and others—rarely—may become cancerous. Both of the latter types require surgical removal.

According to the Thyroid Foundation of America, as many as two million individuals in the United States have undergone childhood radiation treatment involving the head and neck for such conditions as acne, tonsillitis, or chronic ear infection. These people are especially vulnerable to developing thyroid nodules, including cancers. The risk is increased if the person becomes hypothyroid; under those circumstances, increased production of TSH from the pituitary gland may stimulate the development and growth of thyroid nodules and cancers. For these reasons, it is safest to surgically remove any thyroid nodule that is detected.

Substernal Goiter

A single, sizeable thyroid nodule may grow downward as the individual gets older, say, through her sixties. It may extend behind the sternum, or breastbone, resulting in substernal goiter. The condition may cause no difficulties at all, or it may result in a mass of tissues hemmed in by the bone. This may cause troubles in breathing and swallowing, often accompanied by wheezing and a noticeably hoarse voice. The thyroid itself may continue to function normally.

WHAT TO DO ABOUT MULTINODULAR AND NODULAR THYROID

Tests

While your doctor may be content to do nothing if you have a simple goiter and are experiencing no problems, he is likely to want to run a few tests if you have developed the multinodular type, which usually persists. He will be even more interested in staying on top of things if there is thyroid trouble of any sort in your family. Blood tests will establish whether your thyroid is making the right amount of hormone, whether it is working under difficulties, and whether there are any antithyroid antibodies circulating (see "Autoimmune Disorders" on page 31). Blood tests will also pick up other chemicals or organisms that might interfere with the harmonious workings of the gland. For more about the various blood tests and other diagnostic procedures covered here, see Chapter 11.

X Rays and Scans

If a patient exhibits pressure symptoms, getting an X ray is vital; these may consist of a plain X ray, an ultrasound, a CT scan, or a barium swallow. The general size and outline of the thyroid shows up in an ordinary X ray or ultrasound. If a substernal goiter is suspected, a CT scan, which produces cross-sectional images, as though the patient's body were sliced across horizontally, reveals the exact situation at every level. A barium swallow involves taking a photo while the patient is swallowing a liquid that shows up on an X ray. This indicates any area of pressure on the gullet.

To check whether the nodules in a nodular thyroid are producing hormones normally, a special type of X ray is used called a *scintigram*. If there is just one lump, it is especially important to determine what it is. It may be a harmless cyst, an area of overactive thyroid tissue (a "hot spot"), an adenoma (which is an unimportant irregularity), or—least likely—a cancer.

FNA

FNA—fine-needle aspiration—is a quick, painless way of taking a sample of the lump, called a *biopsy*, and then determining with a microscope its exact composition.

Treatment Options

If the tests show that your thyroid is working normally and its size is no bother to you, action may not be needed at present, but you should undergo annual checkups. If antithyroid antibodies are present in the blood, it is particularly sensible to have regular follow-ups. Your hormone production could fall off gradually without your being aware of it, even if it is satisfactory now.

Of course, if you are found to have too much or too little thyroid hormone, your doctor will ask you many more questions and perhaps arrange further tests. Then you will start on specific treatment. This is likely to be medication of whichever kind is appropriate (see Chapters 3, 4, and 11). If, however, your thyroid is too bulky to be elegant and comfortable, if it is causing pressure problems in your breathing or swallowing tubes, or if it has sneaked behind your breastbone, an operation is the quickest, safest, and most effective treatment. There is no medicine that will make an enlarged thyroid shrink when it has become nodular. On the other hand, you will probably need to take thyroxine (synthetic thyroid hormone) indefinitely after the operation. This will not only prevent your running short of the hormone now that you have lost part of the production line, but it will also tend to discourage any propensity in the remaining part to overgrow again.

As mentioned above, when there is a single nodule of any kind—whether a harmless cyst, an overactive hot spot, a tumor, or a substernal goiter—surgery is the best treatment.

> Julie was thirty-eight. She ran the lingerie department of a department store efficiently and seemed generally fit. She had sailed through a recent routine medical examination. Nevertheless, she had one niggling symptom. We all choke at mealtimes occasionally, when something "goes down the wrong way," but it was a regular nuisance for Julie. She also had spells of coughing from time to time, and found she was more comfortable sleeping with three pillows.
>
> Julie consulted again with a doctor, who could find nothing wrong physically. Her thyroid tests were all normal, so the doctor arranged for a chest X ray. It showed a fleshy lump behind the breastbone. A CT scan located it more precisely, and a scintigram showed that it was active thyroid tissue—a substernal goiter. The unwanted part of the thyroid was removed surgically, and the symptoms disappeared. The thin line of a scar at the base of Julie's neck hardly showed, and a necklace hid it completely.

ENDEMIC OR IODINE-DEFICIENCY GOITER

Everything we have discussed so far has been concerned with a healthy thyroid that has grown oversize without any apparent outside cause and that continues to function normally. Various other conditions exist in which the thyroid swells in response to something harmful. In iodine-deficiency goiter, for example, the cause lies within the patient's living environment.

Endemic goiter—so called because it is regularly found in certain regions—is still prevalent in many parts of Asia, Africa, and South America, especially in such mountainous districts as the Himalayas and the Andes. It affects more than three hundred million people in Asia alone. Goiter epidemics used to exist in a few isolated pockets in Europe and North America, but the problem no longer exists in the industrialized countries, apart from certain exceptional circumstances. One such circumstance might include recent immigration to the West from a country with iodine deficiency.

All the places where iodine-deficiency goiters are common are distant from the sea or ocean, the basic source of iodine all over the world. Iodine gets into the soil and water supplies from the wind and the rain off the sea, and from there into the plants, milk, and meat people eat. Besides inland regions, some valleys that were long ago cleared of their topsoil by glaciers have been left bereft of iodine, even near the coast. (The ancients thought the reason some valley-dwelling people developed goiters was because the air was "too concentrated" there.)

With the sophisticated transport and distribution systems we enjoy in the industrialized countries, we get our food from all over the world: bananas from Belize, coffee from Columbia, oranges from Israel, and fish from the sea. In the remote areas of the Thirld World only local produce is available, and its iodine content is dependent on the mineral content of the soil there.

If a Westerner takes a short trip to Tibet or a safari across Africa, he or she may be deprived of iodine. This will not matter; remember the three months' reserve supply stored by the thyroid (see preceding chapter). On the other hand, if you are planning to stay for months or years in a remote mountainous district, it would be wise to find out if goiter is prevalent there. Discuss with an expert the advisability of taking along iodized table salt or some other source of iodine.

If you live in the West, there is more danger of your taking in too much iodine than too little. You cannot get too much from eating a normal diet; the risk lies in taking unprescribed iodine supplements, or becoming a kelp freak. Kelp is a seaweed that is very rich in iodine. It came into vogue as a health food in ancient China, medieval England, and early-twentieth-century America, when goiter was rife in some states, such as Michigan. The thyroid responds to overdosing with iodine either by producing too much hormone or, paradoxically, by stopping hormone production altogether. The gland enlarges either way.

The thyroid gland gets bigger when it has to work extra hard, as in pregnancy. Shortage of iodine—an essential constituent of the thyroid hormones—means that it has to manage under difficulties. In such a case the gland swells up and may become enormous. Early pictures and descriptions of goiter are likely to depict people living in iodine-deficient areas. The Chinese in 1600 B.C. and the Vedic Indians twelve hundred years later found a cure: powdered burnt seaweed, sponge soaked in wine, or powdered mollusk shells. No one knew specifically about iodine until centuries later.

Compared with Asia, Europe was slow to catch on to a cure for goiter, although Hippocrates, circa 400 B.C., noticed the association between goiter and living in the mountains. He put it down to drinking melted snow. The Romans blamed "the noxious qualities of the water" in the Alps. Marco Polo, in his travelogue of 1299, described "tumors of the throat, occasioned by the quality of the water." No cure was mentioned. In England, Shakespeare's Gonzalo, in *The Tempest*, speaks of "mountaineers... whose throats had hanging at them wallets of flesh." In the eighteenth century most of the countries of Europe included particular "goiter areas."

It was not until 1811 that Bernard Courtois discovered violet-colored crystals that he called "Substance X." This was iodine. Over the next fifty years, despite some disastrous mistakes made in figuring out how to use it, iodine came to be the cure or preventive measure for endemic goiter. The Swiss were the first to come up with the idea of putting iodine into the salt people consumed; by 1917, they had eliminated the illness from their country. The Americans adopted the same system soon after, but it was not until 1960 that the British caught up. Nowadays, however, because of the variety of foods generally available in this country, iodization is no longer necessary.

Although lack of iodine in the soil is the main cause of endemic goiter, it is not the only one. The next great discovery about goiter can apply to any of us today. In 1928, Dr. Alan Chesney at Johns Hopkins Medical School realized that something in cabbage was causing his rabbits to develop swellings in their necks. Now we know that the brassica group of vegetables—cabbage, kohlrabi, brussels sprouts, and cauliflower (but not broccoli)—contain goitrogens. These are chemicals that prevent the thyroid from making its hormones in spite of plenty of iodine; they thereby produce an effect similar to that of iodine deficiency.

In the case of brassicas, the goitrogens are cyanide derivatives called *thiocyanates*. They also get into the diet when milk from cows who have been fed kale and raw turnips is consumed. Children in Tasmania started developing goiters through drinking milk from kale-fed cows. This was most noticeable in the spring, when thiocyanate levels in the plants are at their highest. Other plants that have a similar effect include soy, rapeseed oil, and peanuts.

Certain medications can also lead to this type of thyroid swelling. They include

- lithium, used in psychiatric illness

- phenylbutazone, for arthritis

- PAS, for tuberculosis

- tolbutamide, for diabetes

- beta-blockers, for high blood pressure

  ➤ resorcinol, a skin disinfectant

  ➤ steroids

Paradoxically, some iodine-containing medicines may act in the same way, including

  ➤ amiodarone, a heart medicine

  ➤ potassium iodide, an ingredient in some cough medicines

It would require regular use of any of these medicines to have an effect.

The goitrogens are more likely to tip the balance toward putting a strain on the thyroid if a person is already vulnerable. This may be because of the presence in that individual's system of autoimmune antibodies (see below), a diet low in iodine, or a family prone to thyroid problems.

The time-hallowed idea that bad water was a cause of goiter has some basis in fact. In some areas an excess of calcium in the water prevents the proper use of iodine by the thyroid. This is most likely to occur in limestone-rich regions. Pollution with urochrome from urine or sewage can also poison the thyroid and has been responsible for some goiters.

See Chapter 10 for more about foods and medicines that can upset the thyroid, and for a discussion of how to keep the thyroid healthy.

Features of the Endemic Type of Goiter

People of any age can be affected by endemic goiter, but women contract the condition at least twice as often as men. The swelling usually begins uniformly but becomes multinodular; it tends to continue enlarging slowly. Sometimes, although the gland is working as hard as it can under difficult circumstances, it may be unable to make enough T_4 and T_3. In that case, all the symptoms and signs of a shortage of thyroid hormone gradually develop. They often include general sluggishness, weight gain, swollen legs, and thinning hair, but there are many exceptions (see Chapter 3). The changes creep up so imperceptibly that they may well go unrecognized as abnormal and instead be attributed to increasing age.

An even more serious threat arises in pregnancy. While the thyroid may be able to produce all the hormones that the mother needs for herself, it is less likely, working under difficulties, to cope with supplying a fast-growing fetus. In centuries past, in the goiter-prone areas, this resulted in a high rate of birth of cretins—the technical term for people deformed and mentally retarded as a result of prebirth thyroid-hormone deficiency. The children were stunted in every way and grew into thyroid-hormone–deprived adults, so there was a population of many people with goiters, some of whom were retarded, and children who never developed properly.

In 1848, in Chiselborough, a village in Somerset, England, all 540 inhabitants had goiters, many were dull and slow, and twenty-seven had major intellectual handicaps. A combination of goiter-producing factors in the environment was responsible. Luckily, no other place in England was so affected, and by 1871 the disorder had subsided . Such a horror could not strike now. Due to efficient testing of adults who develop goiters and routine thyroid tests for pregnant women and newborn babies, these epidemiological disasters are a thing of the past in our culture. Such conditions should soon be banished all over the world with the spread of medical knowledge and techniques.

Treatment Options

If you are on one of the long-term medicines that can upset the thyroid, it is essential to have regular checkups to make sure that your thyroid is producing adequate amounts of hormone and doing so without serious struggle. The TSH test (see Chapter 11) provides this latter information. You don't want to wait until the symptoms of thyroid-hormone deficiency sneak up on you.

If the tests are normal, you will need no active treatment, but you will require regular follow-up. If your hormone levels are satisfactory but your TSH level is raised, the doctor may put you on a small supplement of iodine and/or a small dose of thyroxine to assist the gland.

You will need special monitoring if you become pregnant (see Chapter 5).

If you test low for the thyroid hormones, the shortfall must be corrected with thyroxine, even if you have none of the indications of underactive thyroid (see Chapter 3).

AUTOIMMUNE DISORDERS

Whereas the most prevalent thyroid problem worldwide is endemic iodine-deficiency goiter, the most common thyroid disorders in the industrialized West result from autoimmune disease. In autoimmunity, the body mistakenly reacts against its own tissues, making antibodies in the blood to fight what it sees as enemies that should not be there, as it would against bacteria, for example. In the case of the thyroid, one or more of several antibodies may be produced against the thyroid's proteins. It is often when the immune system is under attack from a virus, or in some cases from a drug to which it is sensitive, that it overreacts and makes antibodies against friends as well as foes. (On the other hand, it is very rare indeed for the bigger germs—the cocci and bacilli—to infect the thyroid. If this does happen, patients may develop a thyroid abscess, but antibiotics are an effective treatment.)

The propensity to autoimmune disease is a genetic tendency, meaning it runs in families. Twenty to twenty-five percent of the population in the United States are thought to have a genetic tendency to autoimmune diseases. People who develop a thyroid disorder may have relatives with other autoimmune illnesses—for instance, rheumatoid arthritis, insulin-dependent diabetes, or vitiligo (a patchy loss of pigment in the skin)—or may themselves suffer from them. If you are one of those who are especially prone to developing autoimmune problems, such conditions are increasingly likely to emerge as you get older. Your immune system gets less efficient, because it has already had a lot to contend with—childhood illnesses, trips abroad, etc.

In the struggle to keep going in the face of interference by antibodies, the thyroid may react in several different ways, leading to one of the following serious thyroid illnesses:

- Graves' disease (a dramatic type of hyperthyroidism, or overactive thyroid)

- Hashimoto's disease, or chronic thyroiditis (very common, and leading to thyroid failure and hypothyroidism, or underactive thyroid)

- underactive thyroid, with or without goiter

- many cases of "simple" goiter

- de Quervain's thyroiditis

Any of these is likely to be accompanied by a goiter. Apart from certain cases of simple, uncomplicated goiter and de Quervain's disease, although the gland may be enlarged, the main features of the illness are caused by underproduction or overproduction of the thyroid hormones. These conditions are dealt with in Chapters 3 and 4.

De Quervain's Thyroiditis

This disorder was first described by Felix de Quervain in the 1920s, but it was only recognized as an autoimmune illness in 1993. The autoimmune reaction seems to be set off by a virus—sometimes the mumps virus. Like mumps (though it is uninfectious), de Quervain's thyroiditis comes in mini-epidemics. Unlike the slow, painless onset of the other thyroid problems, this comes on very rapidly, with sudden, painful swelling of the gland.

The pain may feel as though it comes from the teeth, the jawbone, or even the ear, but touching the hard, tender thyroid settles the question. It hurts to swallow, laugh, or nod the head, and the patient suffers from headache, aching in the muscles, and raised temperature.

The illness goes through two very different stages, each lasting several months, after the general feeling of acute illness has died down. The first stage is overactivity of the thyroid, when it is reacting with irritation. This results in nervousness, restlessness, and a racing pulse. The second stage is underactivity, when the gland is tired from its exertions. The patient is forced to slow down and feels weary, cold, and constipated.

Treatment Options

No specific medicine exists to deal with the cause of de Quervain's thyroiditis, but there are plenty that will make the patient more comfortable. Steroids such as prednisolone are likely to cut the whole illness short, and patients may find mild painkillers like aspirin or Tylenol helpful for the initial neck pain. Beta-blockers may be required to calm the heart rate and the mind, and possibly a small dose of thyroxine will be prescribed in the final stages. The good news is that in most cases everything returns to normal after the illness has run its course. (By contrast, Hashimoto's underactive thyroid—another of the autoimmune thyroid problems—affects some people long term.)

TUMORS OF THE THYROID

Adenoma of the thyroid—a noncancerous tumor or cyst, like the harmless, lumpy areas in the breast that cause so much needless worry—tends to crop up from around age thirty-five onward. No health risk is involved, but it is usually more comfortable to have the adenoma removed and end any anxiety. Benign tumors are far more common than thyroid cancer.

In the United States, twenty-five people per million develop thyroid cancer each year (six thousand cases), accounting for 0.6 percent of cancers in men and 1.6 percent of cancers in women. No one welcomes cancer, but thyroid cancer has three pluses on its side. First, it causes so little trouble that it is frequently discovered only after the person's death from something quite unrelated. Second, of those that are diagnosed during life, over 90 percent are curable. Third, an effective early-warning system exists in the form of a blood test.

The tumor starts as a lump in the thyroid. That is why any solitary nodule in the gland merits checking out thoroughly, however unlikely it is to be a cancer. This is one thyroid disorder that doesn't run in families, and there is no extra risk if you have a goiter or any other thyroid symptom.

Treatment Options

The cancerous lump is removed surgically, along with as much of the surrounding gland as the surgeon thinks necessary. For some people, radioactive iodine, in the form of a drink or capsules, is given as an extra precaution after surgery. In all cases, replacement therapy with thyroxine tablets is needed indefinitely, to compensate for the loss of thyroid activity.

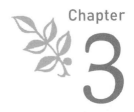

Chapter

3

Underactive Thyroid

The trouble with an underactive thyroid is that you may not know you have one.

An underactive thyroid fails to produce enough of the hormones T_4 and T_3 to meet the individual's mental and bodily needs. The scientific name for this condition is hypothyroidism. *Hypo* is the Greek word for *under*. (Rather confusingly, *hyper* means the opposite; therefore, hyperthyroidism means an overactive thyroid.) Another term still in use for thyroid underactivity is *myxedema*. It was coined by a Dr. Ord in 1877, and it refers to the puffy swelling (*edema*) of the skin that accompanies the condition.

Underactive thyroid is common—probably more so than is recorded—and in some countries its incidence is increasing, especially among elderly women, as a recent study from the United Kingdom indicates. Baseline assessments of thyroid function were made on 2,779 randomly chosen adults of either sex in the Tyne and Wear district of England, and repeated twenty years later on the 1,877 survivors. The women in the study had developed spontaneous hypothyroidism at the rate of 3.5 cases per 1,000 per year, compared with 0.6 cases per 1,000 per year for the men. (There had been no excess of thyroid abnormalities among those who had died.) The average age for the diagnosis of hypothyroidism was fifty-eight or fifty-nine, but the likelihood of developing it increased steadily with age, reaching 14 cases per 1,000 per year for women ages seventy-five or eighty.

In the United States, by some estimates, as many as 8.6 million women suffer from hypothyroidism, with over 80 percent of those going untreated. (The ratio is even worse for men: An estimated 1.7 million American men are hypothyroid, yet only about 100,000, or fewer than 6 percent of them, are getting treated for it.) Like depression, which often accompanies it, hypothyroidism usually creeps up so slowly that you think it's "just you," or "only to be expected at your age."

In 1873, Sir William Gull, Queen Victoria's doctor, who first linked the thyroid with some curious changes affecting mostly women nearing menopause, described one of his patients as follows: "Miss B., after the cessation of the catamenial period [i.e., after the menopause], became insensibly more and more languid, with general increase in bulk. The change went on from year to year, her face altering from oval to round, like the full moon at rising...the voice guttural...the hands peculiarly broad and thick."

Miss B. did not wake up one morning with a swollen face, as one does with mumps. The changes caused by an underactive thyroid are so gradual that the person's family and even her doctor may fail to realize what is happening. Sometimes a new doctor will spot the disorder, as happened with Phyllis.

> When Phyllis was visiting her mother, who was in the hospital with complications from diabetes, she had a chat with the resident. To her surprise, he seemed more interested in her health than in her mother's. He had noticed that Phyllis was plump, a little short of breath, and had some external features indicating hypothyroidism.

Most of us will not find ourselves in circumstances where the queen's doctor or a bright young resident has occasion to cast a clinical eye over us. It is up to us to report to our doctors any changes we experience, including the vague, general ones.

Nowadays, unlike in 1873, it is extremely worthwhile to recognize hypothyroidism as soon as possible, because a definite cure exists. If, for instance, your skin seems slightly thicker and yellowish, you've put on a few pounds without eating more, and everything feels like an effort, don't just assume it's your fault. One reason for the insidious way in which thyroid-hormone-deficiency problems crop up is that the gland struggles to keep going in the face of difficulties, often growing larger with the effort. Another reason is our big reserve store of both iodine and partly manufactured hormones. With this backup supply in place, the thyroid won't one day simply quit working, resulting in a drastic onset of recognizable symptoms; rather, the symptoms emerge gradually and insidiously.

SYMPTOMS

Another factor that allows so many people to slip into hypothyroidism unawares is the extraordinary variety of symptoms it can produce, apparently without rhyme or reason. You can't predict which is likely to affect you, nor in what order. The symptoms fall into three groups: those affecting appearance, physical health, and mental and emotional state.

In addition, but only very rarely, severe, long-term hypothyroidism can result in serious psychiatric disorder, or in a coma. This section describes all of these symptoms.

Appearance

Any of the following signs, in an early stage, may alert you to the possibility of an underactive thyroid. Comparison with a photograph taken a few years earlier can make most changes more obvious.

Face
Full and puffy. The skin looks thick, almost padded—notably the eyelids, especially the lower ones.

Complexion
Pale and porcelain-like from anemia, but with a pink flush over the cheekbones. Alternatively, it might take on a lemony tint. This results from a buildup of carotene in the body, because it cannot be converted to vitamin A without adequate thyroid hormone.

Lips, Tongue
Lips are swollen and pouting, of a purplish hue. The color is caused by poor, slow circulation. The tongue is enlarged and may be more visible than usual.

Eyebrows
The outer third of both eyebrows lose their hair.

Expression
Sad, lackluster.

Head and Body Hair
Becomes scanty and paler. Head hair loses its sheen, causing it to look as though it is dulled by too much hairspray. The hair will not hold a perm.

Skin
Thick, dry, and slightly peeling; cool to the touch. There may be a rash over the body that looks like a reddish network.

Vitiligo
A patchy loss of pigment in the skin, affecting any area of the body and slowly spreading over more of the body and face. It is made worse by exposure to sunlight. Although it looks odd, the skin is perfectly healthy. This is an autoimmune condition.

Nails
They are very slow-growing and develop ridges.

Xanthelasma
Little yellow lumps around the eyes. These are made of cholesterol, and indicate a high level in the blood. They can be a useful

hint to get your thyroid checked; in any case they are a warning to take steps to reduce the fat and cholesterol in the bloodstream.

Hands, Feet, and Ankles
They are enlarged, causing rings and shoes to feel too tight.

Clothes
These are as characteristic as any outward feature of an underactive thyroid. You will be wearing thicker, heavier, woollier garments, and more of them than you did previously.

Physical Health

Heartbeat
The usual effect of hypothyroidism is a slowing of the heart rate, but the heart rhythm may also be affected, particularly in those over fifty. The rate may be as low as fifty beats a minute compared with the usual seventy to eighty. A slow heart rate means sluggish circulation, in turn leading to cold skin, blue lips, ankle swelling, impotence, and a risk of congestive heart problems. An uncorrected high level of cholesterol can result in furred arteries and the possibility of heart attack. Palpitations may occur.

Blood Pressure
May be low because of the slow heart rate, or high because of clogging of the arteries due to excess cholesterol.

Chest Pain
In people with Hashimoto's hypothyroidism (see "Causes of an Underactive Thyroid," below), pain in the front of the chest is common. Angina, on the other hand, is uncommon when there is a low level of thyroid hormones, but if treatment with thyroxine is started too abruptly, the typical chest pains of angina are likely to arise. Anginal pain feels tight and restrictive across the chest when you are walking uphill, but it stops when you stop the exertion. The effect is temporary, but requires a slowdown in building up to the correct dosage of thyroxine.

Shortness of Breath

This is common and has several contributing causes, including increased weight, anemia, slow heart, and collection of fluid in the chest (similar to swollen ankles).

Weight

The most typical change is an increase of, say, ten pounds over a year, despite a decrease, if anything, in appetite. This is due to the slow metabolic rate.

In 1947, Dr. Adolf Magnus-Levy was studying obesity. He gave an overweight nurse extra thyroxine and found afterward that she was using 30 percent more oxygen than before. This meant she was burning up her food faster. From there, Magnus-Levy developed the concept of basal metabolic rate (BMR; see Chapter 1), which is controlled by the thyroid hormones. The nurse had been hypothyroid, and she lost her excess weight gradually when her hormone levels were restored to normal.

Not everyone who is hypothyroid gains weight; some may actually get thinner, because their metabolism is inefficient in its slowness. This "reverse effect" of weight loss can happen at any age but is most common in those over thirty-five.

Another anomaly arising from hypothyroidism that can spoil a person's figure is bloating—a buildup of gas during the day, making the tummy bulge. The problem isn't an excess of body fat, and it may be remedied by a change of diet as well as by thyroid treatment.

Tinnitus

This is an irritating ringing or whistling noise, usually occurring in one ear only. It affects two-thirds of those with an underactive thyroid. Unlike tinnitus resulting from other causes—wear-and-tear or physical damage, for example—this type may improve with treatment.

Hearing Loss

Hearing loss affects about one-third of those with an underactive thyroid. It is caused by a direct effect on the auditory nerves arising from a shortage of T_4 in the nerves. It is seldom severe (individuals affected find that they sometimes miss hearing the telephone, for example), and it gets better with thyroid treatment.

Voice Change

This results from swelling of the vocal cords and of the tongue, and it is most noticeable on the phone. The doctor and philosopher Robert Asher described the effect as "like a bad gramophone record of a drowsy, slightly intoxicated person with a bad cold and a plum in the mouth." In truth, it rarely reaches anything close to that level of severity. You might at first find it rather sexy—your voice is a little deeper and huskier than usual.

Intolerance to Cold

An affected person's internal heating is turned down, so that she feels unpleasantly chilly when everyone else complains of the heat. Her hands and feet are cold, and she is subject to chilblains or Raynaud's disorder. In Raynaud's disorder, the hands turn mottled red and dead white at the slightest coolness and are painful, blue, and swollen when warmed. The sufferer is at higher risk than others of developing hypothermia. Although thyroid treatment will put matters right, it takes several months to do so. During that time, keep your home no cooler than 70 degrees.

Sleep

You miss out on stage-4 sleep, the deepest and most restful type. Loss of deep sleep leaves you tired all day, and sleepy.

Snoring

Your partner will be more aware of your snoring than you are. In any case, it may indicate sleep apnea. Sleep apnea causes breathing to slow down during sleep, and then to speed up again with a jerk that may awaken the sleeper several times a night. She feels unrefreshed and headachy in the morning.

Muscles

In general they very gradually become weaker and stiffer, and they may ache. All of the muscles may be affected, but especially those in the shoulders and thighs. The condition makes it difficult to keep up on a walk.

Cramping Calves

This may occur when you are walking uphill, and it results from poor circulation. Muscle cramps that come on even during rest happen only if the thyroid has been knocked out suddenly—for instance, by an operation, or by radioactive iodine (used to treat overactive thyroid) given without sufficient preparation.

Joints

Like the muscles, the joints may also be stiff and painful. They may be swollen by fluid collecting in them. Joints most likely to be affected are the knees, fingers, wrists, or neck, in combination or individually. Unlike with other forms of arthritis, the discomfort is not usually any worse in the mornings when you first get up. Thyroid treatment is effective, but it may be a year or more before full recovery.

Pins and Needles

There are two ways in which lack of thyroid hormone can cause this odd, unpleasant sensation in the fingers. The most likely is a direct effect on the nerves to the hand, but in about 7 percent of cases this sensation is a symptom of carpal tunnel syndrome. The carpal tunnels are the sheaths that cover the tendons in the wrists, and hypothyroidism may cause them to become swollen, as it does many other body parts. This makes it painful and stiff to move the fingers, as well as causing painful pins and needles.

Dizziness and Poor Balance

These result from impairment of the nerves due to lack of thyroid hormone. The unsteadiness can make you nervous about going out, but if it is a thyroid problem, a remedy exists.

Tremor
Especially noticeable when you pick up a cup or glass full of liquid. Like pins and needles, tremor may result from a shortage of T_4 to the nerves of the hands.

Fainting
Fainting spells result from slow circulation, which leads to low blood pressure.

Menstrual Periods/Bleeding
They often become very heavy, and more frequent as well, but in a minority of cases they stop altogether. There is also a general tendency to bleed for longer than usual if you cut yourself.

Infertility
This is a common effect that can occur in either sex (see Chapter 5).

Anemia
Anemia that accompanies hypothyroidism may be either ordinary iron-deficiency anemia, which is made worse by heavy periods, or pernicious anemia. Like the Hashimoto's type of underactive thyroid (see below), pernicious anemia is an autoimmune disorder, and it may show up before, after, or during hypothyroidism.

Constipation
This is particularly likely to be a nuisance to the older person. The cause lies in the nerves controlling the bowels, which make them work more slowly.

Don't assume that if you are hypothyroid you will exhibit all or even many of these physical symptoms. If one or two of them crop up without an obvious reason, tell your doctor. Lack of thyroid hormones may not be to blame, but it is worth checking out since hypothyroidism can be easily remedied.

With Marion, it was her cholesterol levels that alerted her doctor. The firm she worked for was concerned about keeping its executives healthy. When everyone had to get their cholesterol checked, Marion's was found to be in the risk range. At thirty-five and quite slim, she was shocked by the results. But there were other things. She had been feeling tired for some time and had wondered if it could be chronic fatigue syndrome [CFS], or perhaps it was because her periods had been so heavy lately. Another problem was her stiff, aching neck and fingers, which she attributed to keyboard work.

Thyroid tests showed that Marion was short of T_4, and an examination indicated that the thyroid gland was slightly enlarged. Treatment restored her to the happy, lively, efficient young woman that she was naturally, with no aches and pains.

Mental and Emotional State

In a way, you are lucky if an underactive thyroid brings on physical disorders; it is much easier to identify these and mention them to your doctor than it is to put a finger on vague, intangible, psychological changes. For instance, how do you explain the paradox that, although you long to be warmer, you actually feel generally worse on a lovely hot holiday in a sunny place? This is because the heat lowers your already substandard thyroid production.

Changes in your outlook, feelings, and efficiency that could indicate thyroid-hormone deficiency include the following:

- Sluggishness and apathy. You can't seem to care, even about people, and nothing catches your interest

- Your senses of smell, taste, and hearing are blunted, so much that such pleasures as eating or listening to music are dulled

- A constant feeling of fatigue, although you are doing less than usual

- Drowsiness all day and evening. You never see the end of a television program because you nod off

- Libido—your sexual feeling—is nonexistent, however attractive your companion

- Efficiency is decreased

- Your memory is unreliable, especially for recent events

- Your concentration is poor; you can't cope with reading anything weightier than a magazine or newspaper article

- Decisions are put off. Your mind goes wearily around and around, getting nowhere

- Day-to-day tasks seem overwhelming

- Nothing feels right about yourself or the rest of the world. This is the worst aspect, and you can't shake it off. The two main features are depression and anxiety. Two-thirds of people with thyroid-hormone deficiency suffer from depression, one-third with anxiety, and often the two overlap

Depression includes pervading unhappiness, loss of hope, and the feeling that you are no good. You try to avoid other people and wish you could go to sleep until the nightmare is over. Nothing is enjoyable. Appetite, energy, and sleep are all reduced.

Anxiety results in your feeling agitated, sure something will go wrong, and worried about things you would have taken in stride before. You can't relax, but nor can you get anything done.

Serious Psychiatric Disorder (Psychosis)

Psychosis resulting from hypothyroidism is rare and arises only when someone has been short of thyroid hormone for years. Ultimately, in this situation, the victim may lose contact with reality. She, or less often he, feels puzzled and afraid and thinks that other people are her enemies. Sometimes she believes she can hear them plotting, or she sees people and scenes that come only from her own mind. Her family will find her irrational and odd in her behavior and will realize that she is ill in some way. Thyroid treatment is needed urgently.

Other psychiatric disorders can be involved in hypothyroidism. For example, there is an increased risk of Alzheimer's disease in people whose brains have been starved of T_4 for a long time. Thyroid treatment, as indicated by tests, is both a preventive and in some people a helpful remedy. The improvement sometimes occurs even when there is no positive test or other sign of thyroid-hormone deficiency. Similarly, some depressives with no symptoms of hypothyroidism and who are not responding to antidepressants may recover if thyroid hormone is added.

Myxedema Coma

This dangerous condition is fortunately very rare, but it can be the first event to draw attention to the sufferer's thyroid illness. It is the end result of untreated hypothyroidism that has built up over the years. Independent-minded, elderly women living alone who "don't want to be a bother to anyone" are the most at risk.

A cold snap is often the final trigger. The victim is found ice cold and barely rousable; her temperature may be as low as 77 degrees Fahrenheit, compared with the normal 98.6 degrees. Understandably, the condition is often mistaken for hypothermia. Alternatively, the cause may be some other illness, such as bronchitis or a urinary infection, that creates extra demands for thyroid hormone. Tranquilizers can have the same effect.

Treatment for myxedema coma is needed urgently, and, unlike with hypothermia, more than gentle rewarming is required. Treatment must take place in a hospital and include steroid injections.

WHAT TO DO IF YOU SUSPECT YOU HAVE AN UNDERACTIVE THYROID

If you have even a vague, slight reason for suspecting that you or a member of your family might have an underactive thyroid, consult your doctor about a thyroid check. A simple blood test for serum levels of thyroid hormone is all that is required to start with. Count it as good news if the thyroid turns out to be under-active; it may be that an easy treatment with tablets will revo-lutionize your strength, mental efficiency, mood, and energy. The next step is to find out what is causing the gland to under-function, and then to plan treatment accordingly. For example, if your thyroid is inhibited by some medication you are taking (see "Medicines That Can Cause Problems," in Chapter 10), it is sensible to review the dosage of the drug rather than immedi-ately start taking extra T_4.

CAUSES OF AN UNDERACTIVE THYROID

Hashimoto's Disease

Autoimmune disorder—in particular, a condition known as *Hashimoto's disease* or *Hashimoto's thyroiditis*—is by far the most common reason for underactivity of the thyroid in the industri-alized world. Older women are most susceptible, especially if there is any rheumatoid arthritis, pernicious anemia, or diabetes in their family. The presence of antithyroid antibodies in a blood test is the giveaway, even if there is no visible sign of enlarged thyroid. When hypothyroidism develops apparently out of the blue, it is probably due to an autoimmune reaction; the same is true when it crops up in someone with a simple goiter (see Chapter 2 for more on simple goiter).

Some children with faults in their chromosomal makeup—including those born with Down's, Klinefelter's, or Turner's syndrome—are particularly susceptible to lack of thyroid hor-mone caused by an autoimmune disorder. They blossom with treatment.

Hashimoto's thyroiditis is named after Hakaru Hashimoto. In 1912, the thirty-year-old Dr. Hashimoto studied four middle-aged Japanese women. Each had a firm swelling in the neck and symptoms of sluggishness, weight gain, and dislike of the cold.

Dr. Hashimoto was so diffident about his paper that he sent it to be published in Germany rather than at home in Japan. It wasn't until 1956 that a group of Americans worked out the autoimmune nature of the problem. Hashimoto's was the first illness shown to be caused by the antibodies' turning against the individual's own body tissues.

Hashimoto's thyroiditis is a cause of goiter in children from around age ten, but is much more frequent in adults. Women are affected twenty times as often as men. Usually the attack on the thyroid by the antithyroid antibodies has been going on for many years before it is recognized.

Diana's story is typical. She had "always" had a slight fullness in the neck. Her mother had noticed it when Diana was about eighteen. It did not lessen over the next two or three years, like the ordinary physiological goiter of puberty, but instead increased a little. Her neck otherwise felt soft and normal, and she was perfectly well. When she was approaching age thirty, the mild swelling shrank a little, but the area felt rather tender and uncomfortable. For a few weeks Diana felt generally tense, and then this feeling and the discomfort subsided.

What was happening was that Diana's thyroid was at last reacting to attacks made by the antibodies by becoming inflamed—a condition called thyroiditis. A brief period of thyroid overactivity made her tense and restless. After that, Diana's thyroid swelling, although quite small, felt firm and rubbery to the touch. Scar tissue had formed in it.

Years went by, and Diana remained busy with career, marriage, and children. Then in her fifties she developed various minor health problems. She lacked the energy to do anything about them, and her family wrote her problems off as caused by middle-age. Her "rheumatism," shapeless figure, slight hearing loss, and poor memory, plus an irritating habit of going to sleep in front of the TV and even at the theatre, didn't seem to add up to an illness. But her thyroid had finally been overwhelmed by the enemies from within and could no longer provide an adequate supply of hormones. Diana's doctor was finally consulted when she alarmed her family by fainting a couple of times.

Diana could have had any of the varied symptoms of hypothyroidism. The trick is to be alert to the first hints, and report them to the doctor. This is particularly important if you are aware of having a goiter, even if it is small and insignificant. If it is large, a Hashimoto's goiter often feels oddly heavy in the neck, unlike simple goiter.

Whereas Hashimoto's is the most common cause of damage to the thyroid that prevents its working properly, there are others, discussed in the remainder of this section.

Iodine Deficiency

Iodine deficiency is seldom a problem in the West. For more discussion of the condition, see the preceding chapter.

Surgery

A thyroid operation for any reason may leave the gland depleted of active, hormone-producing tissue. A handful of surgeons in the 1880s noticed that, some time after being operated on for goiter or overactive thyroid, their patients developed what they called *cachexia strumipriva*. The condition comprised the same collection of symptoms as myxedema and was a clue to the connection between myxedema and the thyroid.

Nowadays, surgeons try to leave enough thyroid tissue for it to function, and they also regularly check their patients' blood for adequate amounts of thyroid hormones. About 20 percent of patients need T_4 supplements after surgery.

Radioactive Iodine and Other Antithyroid Drugs

Surgery is no longer the only treatment for an overactive thyroid, but the medicines used instead may be even more destructive of thyroid tissue. Radioactive iodine is an excellent form of treatment, but its effects continue for years after it has dealt with the overactive gland. After one or two decades, between 65 and 70 percent of those given radioactive iodine slip into thyroid-hormone deficiency and need supplemental T_4.

The other antithyroid drugs used to treat an overactive thyroid, such as carbimazole (Neo-Mercazole), methimazole (Tapazole), or propylthiouracil (Propylthiour, or PTU), have a similar effect, but they act more quickly. This unwanted effect is usually reversible if and when the medication is no longer necessary, or fine-tuning may be done by adding thyroxine as necessary. (See Chapters 4 and 11 for more about radioactive iodine and the other antithyroid drugs.)

Less Common Causes

Less common causes of an underactive thyroid include the following:

De Quervain's Thyroiditis
The aftermath of this acute inflammation of the thyroid may be long-term damage to the active tissues. Complete recovery is the more likely outcome, but thyroxine treatment is needed until the gland can once again make enough hormone. (See the preceding chapter for more on this condition.)

Excess Iodine Intake
Individuals can get too much iodine from such medicines as amiodarone and potassium iodide, from overuse of seaweed preparations (common in Japan), or by taking iodine supplements without the doctor's say-so. (See Chapter 10 for more about the sources of iodine.) Excessive iodine can stimulate the thyroid to make too much T_3 and T_4, or, conversely, can inhibit the manufacture altogether.

After Giving Birth
Some mothers develop temporary thyroid failure after giving birth and require treatment while the situation lasts (see Chapter 5).

Lithium

Lithium is taken for an indefinite period as a preventive in some types of psychiatric illness. In over one-third of the people who take lithium, it precipitates the autoimmune reaction called Hashimoto's disease. Affected individuals must take replacement thyroid hormone while a change is made to a different medication for the psychiatric condition.

Other Medicines That Can Impair Thyroid Function

These include phenytoin, sulfonamide, tolbutamide, androgens, salicylates, and steroids. For more about these, see Chapter 10.

Diet

Diet can be harmful to thyroid function in several ways (see Chapter 10):

- goitrogens in the food—contained in vegetables of the brassica family, soybeans, almonds, sweet corn, and milk from animals fed on certain fodder—may inhibit thyroid functioning

- an excess of fiber may cause the bowel to be emptied too soon for sufficient iodine to be absorbed

- a strict salt-free diet may prevent the uptake of iodine

Certain Minerals in Excess

Cobalt, fluorine, calcium, bromine, and nitrates—either from the water supply or from misuse of health foods, medicines, or multivitamin/multimineral pills—can impact thyroid function.

Starvation

Although starvation from any cause can affect thyroid function, the most likely cause of undernutrition in the industrialized nations is anorexia nervosa (see Chapter 7).

Physical Illnesses Unrelated to the Thyroid

Any severe illness, and some that are not particularly severe, can cause an upset in thyroid-hormone production, including:

- Liver disorders such as cirrhosis, physical damage to the liver (as from an accident), and autoimmune liver disease

- Kidney disorders, such as nephrosis or chronic renal failure, which is accompanied by goiter in nearly half the sufferers. A kidney transplant causes the thyroid function to return to normal, but dialysis has no such effect

- Diabetes, but only if poorly controlled, with the occurrence of hypoglycemic episodes

- All cancers, but especially lung cancer

- Autoimmune diseases, especially pernicious anemia, lupus, rheumatoid arthritis, and Addison's disease

Recovery from Surgery and Burns

There is a flash increase in thyroid-hormone production during a surgical operation and a temporary hypothyroid stage during the convalescent period. The same thing happens after a severe burn. Neither case needs treatment.

Drugs

Those who use heroin or methadone illegally and without medical supervision may inadvertantly upset their thyroid.

SECONDARY HYPOTHYROIDISM

All the problems mentioned so far have been caused by the thyroid itself and its reaction to various outside influences. In a few rare cases, however, thyroid-hormone deficiency can occur even though the gland is in perfect working order and there is nothing in the outside environment upsetting it. Such cases arise from faults in the control centers in the pituitary gland and the hypothalamus, which regulate the thyroid (see Chapter 1). These faults are of overriding importance in themselves; any resulting thyroid problems are secondary. A pituitary tumor, probably nonmalignant, is the most common of this rare group of causes.

TREATMENT OF AN
UNDERACTIVE THYROID

In essence, treatment of a thyroid-hormone deficiency could not be more straightforward: simple replacement in tablet form of the missing hormone. This is all that is required in the vast majority of cases, but it is also vital to eliminate or deal with any underlying cause.

In 1891, a London physician named Dr. Murray, who was one of the first to believe that the thyroid affected every part of the body and brain, made a marvellous breakthrough when he cured his myxedematous patient with injections of sheep thyroid. She lived another twenty years, to the age of seventy-four, but it took the thyroid glands of 870 sheep to keep her in good health. The next advance was finding that the extract was just as effective when taken by mouth. On Christmas Day in 1914, another leap forward came when the chemist Edward Kendall discovered how to make pure thyroxine, such as we use today. From that day on, sheep no longer had to be sacrificed and a chemical process was all that was needed. In addition, the product could be given in precise doses.

Although the thyroid produces two hormones—T_4 (thyroxine) and T_3 (triiodothyronine)—replacement of thyroxine alone is all that is required, since the body converts T_4 to T_3 as and when needed, even if the thyroid is underfunctioning. The usual dose of thyroxine ranges between 100 and 200 micrograms (mcg) daily, with proportionately more for children and less for the elderly, based on growth and energy requirements.

Caution: if you are over forty-five or severely hypothyroid, it is important to start treatment with a low dose, say, 25 mcg daily, or to take it on alternate days. Your doctor will increase the dosage in small steps over weeks and months. It is not worthwhile to test your thyroid status until two months after you have started treatment. The dose you and your doctor settle on will depend on how you feel, as well as on blood-test results.

Some people experience harmless palpitations when they first take thyroxine. A small dose of beta-blocker (see Chapters 4 and 11) will tide them over during this uncomfortable phase, which is temporary and not dangerous. Other people endure aching in the muscles, which is also temporary and of no serious significance. Indications that the dose is too high too soon include muscle cramps, angina, shortness of breath, and ankle swelling. If you experience any of these, you and your doctor should continue working to adjust the dose.

There is danger and no advantage in taking more T_4 than the tests and your doctor suggest. Rather like alcohol, the right amount is a good thing, but too much is bad.

In most cases treatment must continue for life and will be monitored from year to year by blood tests. Conveniently, there is no need to take thyroxine more than once a day, and it doesn't matter at what time you take it.

The development of the treatment for underactive thyroid has been very rewarding. Sir William Osler in 1896 was almost lyrical: "[T]hat we can today restore children otherwise doomed to helpless idiocy and that we can restore to life the hopeless victims of myxedema is a triumph of experimental medicine." It is no longer experimental.

SUBCLINICAL HYPOTHYROIDISM

Ordinary hypothyroidism is fairly easy to recognize, and the diagnosis is readily confirmed by blood tests showing a low level of thyroxine in the serum. The condition responds to simple treatment with thyroxine tablets. By contrast, subclinical hypothyroidism, a first cousin to hypothyroidism, presents quite a different matter. The condition has only been recognized in the last few years, but is increasingly common. Five times as many women as men are affected. By the age of fifty, an estimated 10 percent of women in the United States have an increased level of thyroid-stimulating hormone (TSH), a sign of a thyroid in distress. By age sixty, the incidence has risen to 16.9 percent of women.

Subclinical means that the condition produces effects that are not detectable by the usual clinical tests. In the case of sub-clinical hypothyroidism, the condition is similar to but falls short of overt hypothyroidism. The symptoms are not specific, but usually include feeling tired all the time and moderate weight gain. Significantly, and disappointingly for the sufferer, the serum levels of the two thyroid hormones, T_4 (thyroxine) and T_3 (triiodothyronine), show up on tests as normal—that's what makes the condition subclinical. However, the serum level of TSH is raised, as it would also be if there were a shortage of either T_3 or T_4.

Until recently, many people, especially women over forty, felt convinced that they had an underactive thyroid but were told that their test results were normal, with the implication that they were fussing over nothing. Recent research has shown that they were justified after all. In the late 1990s, the TSH test, often the starting point for determining thyroid health (see Chapter 11), was reevaluated. Results greater than 2.0 m-IU/L (milli–international units per liter) are now often regarded as abnormal (in the past the usual cutoff was 4.0 m-IU/L).

A further test showing the presence of antithyroid antibod-ies in the blood adds to the evidence that thyroid function is declining and that a substantial risk exists of the patient's devel-oping full-blown hypothyroidism in the next five years. Over the twenty years following the diagnosis of subclinical hypothy-roidism, the chances of its advancing to fully developed hypo-thyroidism increase steadily, especially once the patient is past age sixty. (There is a high TSH level in some cases of infertility and in most cases of autoimmune disease, but this in itself is not a reliable marker for subclinical hypothyroidism.)

Who Should Be Tested?

Thyroid experts advise TSH screening for women every five

years starting at age fifty, and for men starting at age sixty. Every woman should be tested as early as possible in pregnancy, and members of both sexes should be screened starting at age thirty-five if there is autoimmune disease or thyroid disorder in the family. In addition to regular screening, the symptoms of lethargy, sensitivity to cold, mild weight gain, or just feeling generally under par may be the earliest indications of subclinical hypothyroidism and should be investigated by the TSH and antibody tests.

Screening for subclinical hypothyroidism is also definitely indicated in the following cases:

- after treatment for hyperthyroidism

- if the individual ever received X-ray treatment involving the head and neck, for instance to treat acne, recurrent tonsillitis, or chronic ear infections

- following surgery on the pituitary gland

- when taking lithium or amiodarone

- following a birth, if the mother has previously suffered from thyroiditis

- in cases of infertility

- in persons age forty and over who have persistent, vague complaints such as fatigue without cause

- in persons suffering intractably depressed moods

According to some researchers, screening may also be useful in individuals with breast cancer, dementia, obesity, or where there is a family history of autoimmune thyroid disease.

Causes

Subclinical hypothyroidism often comes on after an episode of excess thyroid hormone (hyperthyroidism or Graves' disease) has been corrected by treatment with radioactive iodine or surgical removal of part of the gland. Ten percent of women in the age bracket fifty-five to sixty who have undergone treatment with radioactive iodine are found to have higher than normal TSH levels. Others develop subclinical hypothyroidism out of the blue. This is particularly likely in those with a tendency to autoimmune diseases, for example rheumatoid arthritis, insulin-dependent diabetes, vitiligo, or pernicious anemia. It is even more likely if blood tests show antithyroid antibodies.

Treatment Options

Unfortunately, treatment for subclinical hypothyroidism isn't as straightforward as treatment for fully developed hypothy-roidism. Most individuals who suffer from subclinical hypothy-roidism, usually middle-aged women, are convinced that they have an underactive thyroid. They persuade their doctors that they need to take thyroxine, and when it fails to solve their prob-lems they want the dosage increased...and increased. The patient and the doctor may wrangle over the diagnosis, with the patient loath to accept that T_4 tablets are not the cure-all they hoped for.

Since 90 percent of sufferers from subclinical hypothy-roidism long to be prescribed thyroxine, and many often feel bet-ter temporarily when they start the medication, several trials have been set up to compare the effects of T_4 with placebo (dummy tablets). In a recent study, 47 percent of those taking T_4 felt better, compared with 19 percent of the placebo patients. This and other studies were conducted using a double-blind for-mat to avoid bias. *Double-blind* means that neither the test sub-ject nor the doctor treating her knows whether she is receiving the real drug or the placebo.

Naturally enough, some victims of subclinical hypothy-roidism are depressed, and doctors have tried giving them T_4 in the hope of improvement, but the results are variable. In patients who have recently been treated for Graves' hyperthy-roid disease, the TSH level fluctuates, making it tricky to assess how much T_4 they need. The worry is that if the dose is too high, the danger of osteoporosis increases, especially in women who are premenopausal. Likewise, too much T_4 can lead to a fast, irregular heartbeat, termed *atrial fibrillation*. In straightforward hypothyroidism there is a rise in the amount of cholesterol in the blood, increasing the risk of coronary heart disease, but it has not been established whether subclinical hypothyroidism has the same effect. Taking T_4 offers the benefit of reducing the serum cholesterol level.

As you can see, the evidence is confusing, but the consensus is that it is wise to take T_4 treatment for subclinical hypothyroidism in order to prevent its developing into full-blown hypothyroidism. If the TSH level is only minimally raised (by less than 0.1 m-IU/L), treatment can be deferred to see if it reverts to normal spontaneously. In any event, cases of subclinical hypothyroidism need long-term monitoring to check for the development of true hypothyroidism.

4

Overactive Thyroid

"A lady, aged twenty, became affected by some symptoms which were supposed to be hysterical...." Dr. Robert Graves was describing a patient in 1835. After about three months she developed a rapid heartbeat and a slight swelling at the front of her neck. These gave him the idea that her problem wasn't "all in the mind." She was, in fact, suffering from an overactive thyroid gland, also called *hyperthyroidism*, meaning "excess of thyroid," or *thyrotoxicosis*, meaning "poisoning by the thyroid."

It was similar for Katie. She was approaching age thirty, and she and Harvey were planning to start a family. They'd had no luck so far, but they'd only been trying for a couple of months. Harvey put her snappishness down to her frustration about not yet being pregnant. Katie had always seemed easygoing, but now she blew up at the slightest thing, and she was so fidgety. Then she made a scene when her mother-in-law made a perfectly harmless remark. Katie decided to ask the doctor for a tranquilizer.

Katie's doctor found that she had a racing pulse and had lost about seven pounds since Christmas, without even trying. Katie was pleased about the weight loss, but went on to explain that she felt worn out for no special reason and wasn't sleeping properly. Routine blood tests traced Katie's problems to an overactive thyroid. Unlike the situation for Dr. Graves' patient, when the only treatment was bloodletting or purging, Katie's doctor was able to offer her a choice of genuine remedies.

An overactive thyroid usually reveals itself faster than an underactive one, but even so it is likely to be several months before the symptoms become so troublesome that the sufferer does something about them. As with most thyroid disorders, women are affected more often than men—in the United States, almost twelve times as many women as men are currently being treated for hyperthyroidism (3,500,000 women to 300,000 men). There is no age limit for the condition in either sex, but it most often strikes those between the ages of twenty and sixty. Individuals who have any autoimmune diseases in their family are especially vulnerable to the most common kind of hyperthyroidism, Graves' disease, named after the doctor mentioned at the beginning of the chapter (see the section on Graves' disease later in the chapter).

Just as in the case of an underactive thyroid gland, it is up to you to be the detective, and to go for a checkup if you get a clue, however offbeat, that your thyroid isn't working properly. The tricky part is that symptoms aren't limited to a single part of the body, but rather can manifest first in any bodily system, including the mind. The medical profession didn't work out the connections between all the many symptoms and an overactive thyroid until well into the twentieth century.

SYMPTOMS

Mood
General nervousness; a mix of anxiety and irritability. You are likely to fly off the handle or dissolve into tears at the drop of a hat. It is like having PMS all the time, only worse, even if you are past menopause. You feel out of sorts but unable to relax, and tired but unable to sleep. You lie awake with thoughts rushing

through your head and your heart thumping, worsened by finding your bed unbearably hot. A few older people don't get the anxious mood; they react to the extra thyroid hormones by an absence of any feeling—complete apathy.

Unfortunately, when it is your spirits and emotions that are most obviously out of order, you are at risk of being written off as neurotic. You are not. To quote an emminent Victorian, an overactive thyroid is a "medical misadventure that might befall anyone."

Tremor

This, too, may be labeled "neurotic," but it is a direct physical effect of the nerves. You may find that your coffee cup trembles embarrassingly, or that your handwriting has become untidy. Even worse is the internal tremor—your body feels trembly and uneasy inside.

Heart and Breathing

Everyone with an overactive thyroid undergoes some change in the action of the heart, and in sufferers over fifty this is usually the most important problem. People of any age are likely to experience palpitations, which manifest as an uncomfortable awareness of the thumping of the heart. The pulse rate may be double its normal pace—at around 150 beats a minute—and occasionally so strong that you can hear it.

The high heart rate and high blood pressure may prevent the blood from returning to the heart efficiently between beats. This leads to swollen ankles and sometimes a collection of fluid in the chest. Since the heart is going at a rapid rate all the time, it cannot speed up when you exert yourself, so you are likely to get short of breath. If you have asthma, it will get worse.

One of my colleagues who prided himself on his squash game was mortified to find that he was losing his edge—at age twenty-nine. He became hopelessly out of breath even when he was playing against his boss, who was quite a few years his senior. It wasn't until he upset everyone by opening all the windows when it was frigid outside that his problem became apparent: He had an overactive thyroid.

Digestive System

Like Katie, you may notice early on that you have magically lost seven to ten pounds, even though you have been eating more than usual. You may also crave those cold, sweet drinks that are so calorie-filled. By contrast, some older people, instead of feeling hungrier, lose their appetite; together with the weight loss, this may make them worry that they have some serious disease.

Bowel movements will be more frequent than usual, and the stool may be pale from the fat being rushed through the intestines before being digested. At the other end, your stomach may be irritable, causing you to vomit easily. This can become an urgent problem.

Skin

You are likely to perspire more, making your skin soft, warm, and damp. The palms of your hands may look flushed, and little spidery veins may appear on your cheeks. The bonus is an ironing out of any wrinkles, but unfortunately this is not permanent. You may feel itchy all over, and hot, so that if you've booked a holiday in the sun you'll wish you were in Iceland.

In some people with the autoimmune type of overactive thyroid, the skin changes color. It may turn a shade darker all over, or, as in Hashimoto's disease, the curious patchy conditon called vitiligo may develop (see preceding chapter).

In addition, two rare skin conditions occur only in autoimmune thyroid disorder. One causes ugly patches of thick red skin to develop over the shins and feet; the other produces a pudgy thickening of the skin on the fingers and feet, making rings and shoes too tight.

The tendency to bruise easily may be caused by the anemia that occasionally develops with an overactive thyroid. If this describes you, tell your doctor, because the anemia may need to be treated separately.

Hair and Nails

Your hair may become extra fine and soft, with an increased tendency to go gray and an obstinate refusal to take a perm. It may also become thinner. (In underactive thyroid the hair also becomes sparse, but it is coarse and brittle.)

A curious sign of overactive thyroid is a partial loosening of the nails, so that the tips ride up slightly and easily catch, for example on your stockings when you are pulling them on.

Neck

Your thyroid gland may look and feel larger to you or to your doctor. Conversely, it may not be swollen at all if, for instance, the problem is too big a dose of thyroxine by mouth.

Muscles and Joints

An excess of thyroid hormone circulating in the body tends to speed up the normal breaking-down of the muscle fibers to a rate faster than they can be replaced. The muscles become weaker; this is especially noticeable in the thighs and shoulders.

Frozen shoulder, often on both sides, is common in hyperthyroidism. The painful stiffness is due to inflammation of the covering of the shoulder joint. Sometimes a shoulder-hand syndrome sets in: Besides the stiff shoudlers, the hands may be swollen and painful. Other joints are not affected.

It may seem surprising that antithyroid treatment helps this kind of problem, especially when similar symptoms in people with an underactive thyroid respond to the opposite treatment.

Libido, Sexual Function, and Fertility

You may find that you've lost interest in sex, but this isn't permanent. Men who are affected by hyperthyroidism may be unable to raise an erection. For women, the condition results in scanty periods or perhaps none at all. If you've stopped menstruating, you might wonder if you are pregnant, but in fact you are unlikely to conceive. If you do, there's an increased risk of miscarriage. For either sex, fertility is reduced.

Eyes

Although they are by no means inevitable, eye symptoms are a particular characteristic of an overactive thyroid. Unlike with most other thyroid symptoms, men are more susceptible to thyroid-related eye problems than women, and so are smokers of either sex. Oddly enough, the eye problems can begin either months before any of the other symptoms or at the height of the illness, or after everything else has recovered. In most cases both eyes are affected, but the symptoms are mild. They amount to a gritty feeling, as though sand has blown into the eyes, and a feeling of discomfort in bright sunshine.

You may notice in a mirror, or a friend may point out, that your eyes look as though they are staring in amazement all the time. They seem bigger because the lids are drawn back and more of the white part shows.

In the autoimmune type of hyperthyroidism, Graves' disease (as occasionally in Hashimoto's disease; see Chapter 3), more serious eye changes may occur. Inflammation of the tissues behind the eyes pushes them forward. This is called *exophthalmos* (another name for Graves' disease is *exophthalmic goiter*). The swelling from the inflammation interferes with the drainage of tears, causing the eyes to water, the upper lids to become puffy, and bags to form under the lower lids. Because of weakened eye muscles, affected individuals may find it difficult to look up, which is tiring. They may also ache all around the eyes. At worst, without treatment there is a risk to one's sight.

The eyes react badly to sudden changes, so treatment of the thyroid problem has to be started gently and carefully. (See Chapter 11 for more on treating thyroid-related eye problems.)

WHAT TO DO IF YOU SUSPECT YOU HAVE AN OVERACTIVE THYROID

The most common symptoms of overactive thyroid are a rapid heartbeat, weight loss, and a swelling in the front of the neck.

There's no guarantee that you'll experience any of these, and to add to the confusion, any one of the problems described in this chapter can be caused by a nonthyroid disorder that may be important or may be trivial. What is certain is that an untreated overactive thyroid is dangerous. Before effective treatment existed, 25 percent of sufferers died. If you suspect that your thyroid could be out of order, see your doctor.

Your doctor will conduct a thyroid check, which consists of a physical examination and a blood test. The physical includes assessment of any thyroid enlargement, looking for skin or eye problems, and checking for tremor in your outstretched hands or your tongue. The doctor will count your pulse and listen to your heart, and may also listen with the stethoscope to your thyroid for an abnormal sound called thyroid bruit (see page 69), and will test your reflexes, which are likely to be quick and jumpy.

The essential adjunct to a physical examination is a blood test to measure thyroid hormones. Other investigations are usually needed only in special circumstances. They include testing for antibodies, X ray, scintigram, electrocardiogram, and measuring the protrusion of the eyes (see Chapter 11 for discussion of these procedures).

If the examination indicates hyperthyroidism, the next step is to decide why.

CAUSES OF AN OVERACTIVE THYROID

An overactive thyroid may be caused by faulty antibodies (i.e., an autoimmune disorder), as is the case in

* Graves' disease

* toxic multinodular goiter (overactive lumpy thyroid)

* toxic nodule (one overactive lump)

* hashitoxicosis (a stage in some cases of Hashimoto's disease)

‣ a stage in de Quervain's thyroiditis

Other causes include

‣ an excess of iodine

‣ an excess of thyroid hormone by mouth

‣ T_3 toxicosis, due to an excess of T_3 (rather than T_4)

‣ disorder of the pituitary gland

‣ cancer

These different types of overactive thyroid require different management, and so do particular groups of people who exhibit any of the conditions, such as

‣ pregnant women and new mothers (see Chapter 5)

‣ babies (see Chapter 6)

‣ children and adolescents (see Chapter 7)

‣ people over fifty (see Chapter 8)

The rest of this chapter is devoted to providing a general overview of the above causes of hyperthyroidism and their treatment options.

GRAVES' DISEASE

Hyperthyroidism may have different characteristics in the young, the elderly, and women who have just had a baby, but the most common cause in all cases is Graves' disease. Ninety percent of thyroid overactivity is caused by rogue antibodies, and three-quarters of this autoimmmune disorder is caused by Graves' disease. The disease is named after Dr. Robert Graves, the Dublin physician mentioned at the beginning of the chapter. He treated three women patients who each had a swelling in the neck and experienced "violent palpitations." Graves wasn't the first to describe the condition—it has also been called Parry's,

Flajani's, and Basedow's disease—but his was the name that stuck.

Dr. Caleb Parry gave a dramatic account of an event that occurred in 1786: "Elizabeth S., aged 21, was thrown out of a wheelchair in coming fast down a hill...and was very much frightened though not much hurt. From this time she has been subject to palpitations of the heart and various nervous affections. About a fortnight after, she began to notice a swelling of the thyroid gland."

Apart from the swelling in the thyroid, which may not always be noticeable, today we would probably put Elizabeth's problems down to PTSD (post-traumatic stress disorder), characterized by anxiety following exposure to an overwhelming, traumatic event. The idea that serious stress can stimulate thyroid overactivity was generally accepted until well after the Second World War. It seemed to be confirmed by a Danish experience. During the German occupation from 1942 to 1944, the annual number of new cases of hyperthyroidism in Denmark jumped by 300 percent; the incidence reverted to the prewar norm in 1945.

In 1956, Hashimoto's disease, the leading cause of underactive thyroid (see Chapter 3), was recognized and proved to be caused by antibodies made in error by the immune system. Only a year later it was established that Graves' disease was produced in a similar way, but with different antibodies, including one known as *TRAb*. The long-accepted theory that an emotional shock or severe, persistent stress bore a direct effect on the thyroid was discarded as superstitious nonsense. Since then it has become clear that it is the immune system that is thrown out of whack by emotional upset, for instance, bereavement.

Now it seems that stress is one of the triggers of the autoimmune process responsible for Graves' disease. Only certain people are susceptible. For example, those affected are likely to have a particular type of tissue, called *HLA-DR3*, as part of the biological makeup they inherited through the genes. That is why a propensity to Graves' disease and other autoimmune problems runs in families. The other autoimmune disorders that may be associated with Graves' disease include

* vitiligo—a patchy loss of skin pigment

* pernicious anemia—a weak state of the blood connected with lack of vitamin B-12

* rheumatoid arthritis—especially in the fingers and knees

* type-I diabetes—an inability to produce insulin, the hormone that controls sugar levels in the blood

* Addison's disease—a disorder of the adrenal gland, leading to general weakness

* lupus—a disorder resulting in episodes of inflammation in joints, tendons, and other connective tissues and organs, and commonly causing skin rashes

* polymyalgia rheumatica—involving severe pain and stiffness in the muscles of the neck, shoulders, and hips

* giant cell (temporal) arteritis—a painful disorder involving inflammation of the large arteries and usually affecting the temples

* myasthenia gravis—a rare, severe muscle weakness

* dyslexia—a reading or spelling difficulty, often involving transposing of letters

If you or members of your family have any of these problems, you are more susceptible to Graves' disease. If any relative has Graves' disease, that increases the risk even more—up to 50 percent if it is your identical twin. If you are female, you run ten times the risk of a male. Graves' disease can crop up at any age from five upward, but is especially likely around age forty—usually before forty in the United Kingdom, and after forty in the United States.

Since you cannot change your sex or genetic makeup, nor escape the unexpected disaster, there are no specific precautions you can take to avoid Graves' disease. However, you can look after your general health and report any doubtful symptoms promptly (see Chapter 10 for advice on how to keep your thyroid happy).

Making Sure It Is Graves' Disease

Listed below are the special characteristics a doctor will look for to distinguish Graves' disease from other forms of hyperthyroidism:

- The thyroid gland is always swollen, perhaps so slightly that the patient doesn't notice it herself. It feels smooth and fleshy, and equal in size on both sides

- Sometimes the gland is so active that it requires a greatly increased throughput of blood. If a doctor listens through a stethoscope, he or she will hear a soft "shush-shush" sound. This is called *thyroid bruit*, and it doesn't occur in any other condition

- A racing heart, of which the patient is conscious, is always present

- Jumpiness, anxiety, and jangled emotions trouble 99 percent of Graves' disease sufferers

- Tremor is almost as common

- Serious eye symptoms and patches of thickened red skin on the shins and fingers crop up less often, but these symptoms only occur in Graves' disease

Tests That Confirm the Diagnosis
Usually all that is needed is the standard "thyroid screen" of blood tests, but additional antibody tests can be made, and a

scintigram shows if the gland is very active all over (see Chapter 11 for more about these and other thyroid tests).

Treatment Options

If Graves' disease has been confirmed as the cause of your problems, this is the go-ahead to start treatment. In general, you need plenty of rest and nourishing food, and you and your doctor will decide together which of the specific treatments is best for you. This depends on your age, sex, the size of the goiter, and your personal circumstances. A number of choices are available. First, there are two types of short-term treatment for swift relief of symptoms: beta-blockers and iodine drops or tablets.

Beta-Blockers

These medicines, of which the best-known is propranolol, are often used to treat high blood pressure. They slow down the heart (relieving palpitations), reduce perspiration, stop tremor, and reduce anxiety. They are taken two or three times a day, or once a day in a long-acting tablet.

Beta-blockers are a useful general-purpose starting treatment, since they act quickly and do not stay too long in the system after treatment ends. The downside is that they have no curative effect; they merely suppress some of the symptoms. Additionally, people with asthma must not take them, and stopping treatment requires tailing off gradually.

Iodine Drops or Tablets

Treatment with iodine in drop or tablet form switches off excess thyroid activity within a few days, but the effect wears off in about three weeks. This treatment is used mainly in preparation for a thyroid operation.

The longer-term curative treatments for Graves' disease include the following:

Antithyroid Drugs

These have a two-fold beneficial effect: They interfere with the overproduction of thyroid hormones, and they suppress the underlying autoimmune process. The best known are carbimazole (Neo-Mercazole), methimazole (Tapazole), and propylthiouracil (Propylthiour, or PTU), the first being more popular in the United Kingdom, and the last in the United States. Whichever you are on, it takes two or three weeks to work, and while you are on it, you need to get regular checkups from your doctor. The dosage of the medicine will vary with the severity of the illness and its progress. If the antithyroid drug is pushing you toward making too little T_4 and T_3, it is usually better to make up the deficit with thyroxine tablets rather than try to get the antithyroid dosage exactly right.

Most people have to stay on antithyroid medicine for eighteen months to two years, after which there is a 40 percent likelihood of a permanent cure, but your doctor may decide to try stopping treatment any time after six months. Your thyroid may have settled back to normality, but if the symptoms creep back after a month or two, it is no good going back on the medicine; you would be certain to relapse again.

Antithyroid tablets are the best treatment for children and adolescents who are still developing, and they are often tried in young women up to the age of forty, but they cannot be taken in the last month of pregnancy or during breast-feeding. For those in whom antithyroids fail to produce a cure, two major treatments are available: radioactive iodine and surgery.

Radioactive Iodine

This is the treatment of choice for an overactive thyroid. Iodine that has been made radioactive is taken up by the thyroid cells just like ordinary iodine, so its radioactive effect is concentrated in the gland. It was first used to cure Graves' disease in 1940—a bonus from the research toward the atomic bomb. Radioactive iodine soon became the most popular treatment for overactive thyroid and has remained so. It is taken by mouth in capsule form, usually one time only. The thought of swallowing something radioactive sounds alarming, but over the last fifty years radioactive iodine has proved safe as well as effective. The only ill effect is a slight soreness in the neck for the first few days.

The only precautions a person who has undergone treatment with radioactive iodine needs to follow are for the sake of other people, and they are temporary. The radioactivity that is not taken up by the thyroid will be eliminated in the urine, mainly in the first two or three days, but until then the patient must keep her distance from other people. That is, don't spend hours in close proximity to another adult, especially someone younger than forty, for instance in bed. You need to sleep in a separate room from your spouse or partner for a couple of weeks. For up to fourteen days (you will be told precisely how long), don't kiss anybody, and don't get nearer than two yards to babies and children. Travelling by public transportation is all right, but postpone any long journeys by car for a couple of weeks. After this period is over, you needn't worry about radioactivity anymore. The exception is if you're considering pregnancy: It is best postponed for six months after taking the dose. Likewise, pregnant women should avoid this treatment (see Chapter 5).

The beneficial effects of radioactive iodine are permanent, but they don't come on full strength for about three months. A beta-blocker is a handy way of keeping comfortable in the meanwhile. Over the ten to twenty years following treatment with radioactive iodine, a fair chance exists that the thyroid will become underactive. This condition is easily put right with thyroxine tablets. In such a case patients don't have to wait for any of the symptoms of thyroid-hormone deficiency to develop; tests done at the annual follow-up will give the doctor advance information, and treatment can be started in good time.

Surgery

An operation to remove part of the thyroid gland is the other choice for a permanent cure. It can be dangerous to operate on an overactive gland, however; it needs to be quieted down first. Beta-blockers only suppress the symptoms—a fast pulse, for instance—but iodine and antithyroid medicines both act directly on the thyroid. For the best results, patients take an antithyroid for a month, to which iodine is added for the last ten days before the operation.

Most people nowadays opt for treatment with radioactive iodine, but surgery is the treatment of choice if you have an unsightly goiter or uncomfortable pressure symptoms, or if you are allergic to antithyroid drugs. You may also choose an operation if you think you might be pregnant, or if you're trying to get pregnant (see Chapter 5).

The operation involves about a week's stay in the hospital. It leaves a small scar, usually hardly noticeable and easily covered with a necklace, scarf, or high collar.

Special Areas of Treatment

Eye Problems

The mild eye discomfort that can accompany Graves' disease normally settles with soothing hypromellose drops (usually called "artificial tears" in the United States) and the use of dark glasses—and of course not smoking, at least until the thyroid itself has recovered. Troublesome eye symptoms may also improve if a beta-blocker is added to other treatment. Although most eye problems improve in step with the thyroid itself, sometimes the timing seems unconnected. If you are unlucky enough to develop very protruding eyes, besides experiencing discomfort, you may see double. Steroid medicines are helpful for this situation, and if all else fails, cosmetic-type surgery or the more recently introduced radiation therapy can put matters right.

Thickened Patches of Skin

These may feel heavy, itchy, and irritable, but the main problem is that they make the legs or hands ugly and misshapen. The most effective treatment is a steroid cream applied at night and worn under a barrier bandage, which is something like plastic wrap. Achieving a cure requires persistence and patience, for it may take over a year.

TOXIC MULTINODULAR GOITER

Toxic multinodular goiter, another autoimmune overactivity disorder, is the second most common cause of hyperthyroidism, accounting for 14 percent of cases. Like Graves' disease, it affects many more women than men, but usually later in life, often at around age sixty.

In toxic nodular goiter, one or more nodules in the thyroid produce too much thyroid hormone. These overfunctioning nodules are actually benign tumors. Toxic *multi*nodular goiter, as its name implies, involves mulitple nodules, giving the thyroid a lumpy consistency. It differs from the type of multinodular goiter covered in Chapter 2 in that it causes the thyroid to overfunction, whereas in "regular" multinodular goiter, the thyroid otherwise functions normally.

> Rita was typical. She'd had a mild fullness of the neck ever since she was eighteen. It wasn't unsightly and hadn't caused her any trouble. She had lived in a rural area for a large part of her early life, and she thought she'd noticed one or two neighbors with goiters. Possibly there was a shortage of iodine or an overabundance of lime in the region. As Rita got older her thyroid became lumpy or nodular, as commonly happens, but she was perfectly well until she was approaching retirement from her job with the electric company. Apparently without rhyme or reason, she developed conditions that her husband attributed to delayed effects of menopause. She was too hot, easily got winded, her hair began to go gray, and she wasn't her usual placid self. She went to the doctor to ask

about hormone replacement therapy, and that was when the real problem was discovered: toxic multinodular goiter.

Because of the age group affected, toxic multinodular goiter frequently leads to symptoms of strain on the heart: shortness of breath, swollen ankles, and disruption to the rhythm of the heart. This last symptom may develop into the rapid irregularity called *atrial fibrillation* (see Chapter 8). Any of the other symptoms of overactive thyroid can, of course, also arise.

Tests

Blood tests show an increase in thyroid hormone, but not as much as in Graves' disease. A scintigram shows some lumpy areas working normally and others doing nothing. An electrical tracing of the heart's action—an electrocardiogram—may be done to provide exact information (see Chapter 11 for more about these tests).

Treatment Options

The same treatments are available as for Graves' disease (see preceding section):

- *Beta-blockers* alone are not enough, but they take the edge off the discomfort for starters

- *Antithyroid drugs* are ineffective; relapse is inevitable

- *Radioactive iodine* would probably be the first choice, unless the goiter is big, ugly, or awkward, in which case *surgery* would be preferred. With this disorder a second dose of radioactive iodine is required in 25 percent of patients, but on the positive side there is less likelihood of promptly developing thyroid-hormone deficiency

Special treatment may be necessary to address heart and circulatory problems. These problems and treatments are dealt with in Chapter 8.

TOXIC NODULE

A solitary "hot spot" is ten times more likely to occur in a woman than in a man, and is usually found in the over-forty age range. The nodule may have been present for a long time, as with multinodular goiter, but a single lump, whether overactive or not, is more likely to be noticeable. A large nodule is more likely to become overactive than a smaller one; hot nodules often measure about one to one and a half inches across. The rest of the gland shrinks and produces no hormone if one part is making too much hormone; this reduces the severity of the symptoms, as compared with Graves' disease or multinodular overactive thyroid.

Tests

- *Blood tests* for hormones usually show an increase in T_4 and T_3, but occasionally in T_3 only

- A *scintigram* usually dramatically pinpoints a hot nodule, but in 5 to 10 percent of cases the overactive part doesn't show up

- *Fine-needle aspiration*, followed by a *biopsy*, is the definitive test. A very fine needle is used to obtain a minute sample of tissue from the nodule. The patient hardly feels anything. The advantage of this test is the precise information it offers, as well as elimination of the possibility that the lump is cancerous

See Chapter 11 for more on each of these tests.

Treatment Options

As with toxic multinodular goiter, beta-blockers are useful only temporarily, and antithyroid drugs are ineffective for the long term.

- *Radioactive iodine* will knock out the overactive nodule, and the rest of the thyroid will gradually recover and resume normal production

- *Surgery* is the treatment of choice if the lump is unsightly or feels like it is in the way, or if the doctor has reason to think that it could become cancerous. Some evidence indicates that having undergone X rays of the head and neck area early in life may make the gland more susceptible to cancer

HASHITOXICOSIS

In a minority of people in the early stages of Hashimoto's disease (see Chapter 3), some of the symptoms of thyroid *over*activity flare up for a few weeks, a condition known as *hashitoxicosis*. These symptoms may be the first indication the patient has of anything wrong, or she may merely be aware of a small goiter of rubbery consistency. She starts feeling ill, losing weight, and suffering from looseness of the bowels. She is aware of palpitations and of feeling overheated.

Tests

The giveaway is the presence of antithyroid antibodies in the blood. Later in Hashimoto's disease, the level of these antibodies sinks to an undetectable level.

Treatment

Treatment is best kept simple, since it will probably not be needed for more than two months maximum. Beta-blockers will help the patient through this period.

DE QUERVAIN'S THYROIDITIS

This painful goiter, discussed in Chapter 2, involves an early stage of overactivity of the gland, leading to the characteristic hyperthyroid symptoms. This stage may last for several months and calls for the use of beta-blockers in addition to treatment for the inflammation.

AN EXCESS OF IODINE

It must have seemed like a wonderful breakthrough when in the nineteenth century it was discovered that a lack of iodine was the cause of the goiters, myxedema, and cretinism common in many areas at that time. Doctors and public-health officers enthusiastically added iodine to flour, table salt, and water. A lot of people were made really ill by overdosing with iodine— notably in Switzerland, a mountainous country with a reputation for goiter.

In some people the reaction of their thyroid to all this iodine was underactivity. Others, more dangerously, were precipitated into toxic overactivity. Nowadays such mistakes concerning iodine quantity seldom occur because we are aware of the dangers of excess iodine. It is unusual for anyone to become ill from an excess of iodine, although there was a recent outbreak in Tasmania—an iodine-containing disinfectant had been used to clean milking utensils.

A person is more likely to have a toxic reaction if she already has a goiter, or if she lives in an area where the normal diet is low in iodine—for instance, in Tuscany or parts of Germany.

Present-Day Sources of Extra Iodine

1. *Radiographic contrast media*: Chemicals used in special X-ray investigations, often of the kidneys or gallbladder

2. *Iodine tincture or powder*: Used to disinfect extensive wounds or burns

In both of the above instances any toxic effects are delayed until several weeks later, because the gland takes time to convert the excess iodine into excess hormone.

3. *Kelp*: A seaweed available in various forms in natural-food stores. Taken to excess it provides too much iodine for the thyroid to cope with

4. *Potassium iodine*: An ingredient in some cough mixtures, which could build up and cause trouble if taken over a long period

5. *Betadine*: Used in mouthwashes. Too much iodine may be absorbed

If iodine overload is suspected or confirmed, any of the above offending chemicals can be discontinued. While the excess iodine is being processed by the thyroid, patients may experience such symptoms as palpitations and overheating; a beta-blocker will tide them over during this limited period

6. *Amiodarone*: This medicine (trade name Cordarone) can be more of a problem. It is an excellent regularizer for disorders of the rhythm of the heart, and usually needs to be taken indefinitely. The daily dose provides a hundred times as much iodine as a normal diet. In most cases the symptoms of overproduction of thyroid hormone don't appear until the person has been on the drug for around thirty to thirty-six months. Then the symptoms come on suddenly. Men are more likely to be affected by hyperthyroidism from amiodarone than women; the drug may cause their original heart-rhythm problems to worsen

It may be unsafe to stop taking amiodarone, and in any case it remains in the system for about a month after the last dose. Beta-blockers and antithyroid drugs are usually given, but the latter take a particularly long time to have an effect. Radioactive iodine is useless, since the thyroid is already as full as it can be of ordinary iodine. Sometimes surgery is the only possible treatment, if the amiodarone must be continued.

AN EXCESS OF THYROID HORMONE TAKEN BY MOUTH

Ingesting an excess of thyroid hormone can occur as a result of the following scenarios:

1. Misjudgement of the dose of T_4 (thyroxine) taken as treatment for underactive thyroid, usually through failing to arrange regular blood tests

2. A vain attempt to cure "metabolic insufficiency," in the belief that it must be due to lack of thyroid hormone

3. The mistaken use of thyroxine to reduce weight

> Charlotte weighed 210 pounds and looked fat. She was fifty and fed up with being overweight. She pressured two separate doctors into prescribing her T_4 and took double doses, hoping to speed up her metabolism and "burn off" the unwanted fat. Instead, her appetite increased, causing her to put on another fifteen pounds. Then she had a minor heart attack.

Thyroid hormones are useless as a slimming aid, because taking the extra hormone switches off the body's own thyroid-hormone production. And as Charlotte's case highlights, doing so can be harmful to the heart and blood pressure.

All that needs to be done to remedy this cause of hyperthyroidism is to cut out or reduce the amount of thyroid taken by mouth, and to monitor the blood level for as long as the doctor advises.

DISORDERS OF THE PITUITARY GLAND

The pituitary gland, located in the brain, produces TSH—thyroid-stimulating hormone. In the rare event of a pituitary tumor, it may make too much TSH and overstimulate the thyroid. Treatment in such a case focuses on the pituitary rather than on the thyroid.

CANCER

Cancer of the thyroid is uncommon, and it is extremely rare for it to cause thyrotoxicosis. Either a large dose of radioactive iodine or surgery—or a combination of the two—is the best treatment for thyroid cancer.

Rarely, a tumor of the testis or of the ovary may lead to symptoms of overactive thyroid. As with pituitary tumor, it is most important to treat the underlying disorder, but a beta-blocker to address the thyroid symptoms may make the patient more comfortable in the meantime.

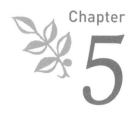

5

Thyroid Issues Affecting Fertility and Pregnancy

"Oh, my throat has come to be swollen," so murmured the beauty. Fearful. Quiet, my child, peace, and hearken to me: "You have been touched by Venus's hand; softly she tells you..."

— Goethe, *The Four Seasons*, 1790

Having a baby—it's the essence of being alive, the most fundamental experience of all. No one who wants it should miss it. A woman's thyroid plays a key role from before conception to after the birth.

> Rob and Vicky had fixed up their home to perfection and made the last payment on their car. Vicky stopped taking the pill and started window-shopping at the maternity stores. After six months: nothing. Vicky's mother and the doctor both said it was still early, so they continued trying. They'd always had a good sex life, but now Vicky found she couldn't summon up any enthusiasm. Her periods were a nuisance, too—heavier than before, and irregular. She blamed them for feeling washed out.
>
> A thyroid test showed that Vicky had an underactive thyroid. She was prescribed thyroxine tablets, and three months later she became pregnant.

FERTILITY

For a member of either sex who wishes to be a parent, a normally working thyroid gland is essential for fertility.

Underactive Thyroid

The symptoms of an underactive thyroid come on so gradually and seem so unimportant at first—slowing down a little, mild weight gain, constipation—that it's not surprising they are often overlooked. Sometimes it is only because of investigations for infertility that the true problem shows up.

The Man's Situation

A man with an underactive thyroid may show an abysmal lack of sexual interest, have a low sperm count, and, at worst, suffer from impotence. This is not a life sentence; normal feelings, function, and fertility are rapidly restored with thyroxine treatment.

The Woman's Situation

As happened with Vicky, an underactive thyroid means loss of libido, plus menorrhagia (heavy menstrual periods), with an underlying failure to ovulate. Sometimes, however, the periods stop, and the woman's hopes are raised that she is pregnant. Treatment is effective.

Overactive Thyroid

Hyperthyroidism can be another cause of infertility. An overactive thyroid is harder to ignore than an underactive one, and treatment is necessary for health and comfort, since the resulting anxiety, restlessness, and palpitations interfere with normal living.

The Man's Situation

Fertility is certainly reduced, but sexual interest and performance may either remain normal or fall off. In some men a swelling of the breast area occurs, and a few are impotent.

The Woman's Situation

Periods are infrequent and scanty, and may cease altogether. Even before this occurs, ovulation (the monthly release of an egg for possible fertilization) is suspended, so conception is unlikely. If a hyperthyroid woman does become pregnant, there is a high risk of miscarriage.

If infertility is caused by either an underactive or an overactive thyroid, treatment of the thyroid problem automatically corrects the infertility. If pregnancy is possible, a woman with an overactive gland must observe special precautions regarding the type of treatment she undergoes. See pages 89–90 for details.

HOW THE THYROID FUNCTIONS DURING PREGNANCY

The thyroid is a vital ally in the whole project of being pregnant. It enables your body to function as usual for ten months, while providing for the total support of a new human being inside you. It stimulates and directs the baby's overall growth, with particular relevance to his or her mental development in the last six months.

If your thyroid is functioning well, you may still feel a bit off for the first few weeks of pregnancy while your system adjusts, but after that, thanks to the thyroid, how you feel during pregnancy is 90 percent positive:

- You don't feel the cold, although heat may begin to bother you toward the end of your pregnancy

- Your circulation is better than usual

- You look well

- You have a good, but not excessive, appetite, and a good digestion to go with it

- You put on weight, but during this period of time you don't have to cut down on your favorite foods

- ⚹ Your mood shifts gradually toward greater optimism

- ⚹ If you have any autoimmune problems—for instance rheumatoid arthritis—they improve

- ⚹ Your thyroid gland, which is working hard, may get a little bigger and feel warm to the touch

The essential factor guiding your physical and mental conditions during pregnancy is your metabolism—the rate at which you burn up your food. By the last few months it will be running at 15 percent above normal. Your heart beats faster and more strongly, and because you are using more oxygen, your breathing is quicker and deeper. There is more blood in circulation, with a generous flow through the uterus and the thyroid. In fact, the output from the heart increases 30 to 40 percent by the twenty-seventh week of pregnancy, though after that it settles down to a slower, steady rate until the birth. These last weeks are important for the subtle and far-reaching developments taking place in the baby's nervous system and brain.

You will be eating a little more, but the increase doesn't amount to "eating for two." Your body's improved efficiency easily provides for bodybuilding—the baby's and yours. Her or his weight increases from zero to six or more pounds, and your weight may climb by as much as seventeen pounds. A large proportion of this is fluid: the baby's water cushion of amniotic fluid, your extra blood, and an increase in body water. In addition, there is development of the breasts (an increase of about two pounds); the uterus itself; and the placenta, through which the baby receives nutrients. There is also a small fat reserve all over the body, but especially in the hips, thighs, breasts, and abdomen, to allow for breast-feeding later.

Not only are thyroid hormones involved in all this construction work—for they are vital in making new protein—they must enable your metabolism to provide you with extra energy. Your muscles have a heavier load to carry, and there is a bigger body to nourish and keep going.

During the first twelve weeks the fetus has no thyroid gland and is entirely dependent on you for his or her thyroid hormone. After that he or she is able to produce most of the necessary supply, but needs a 20 percent top-off from you.

Thyroid Tests

Thyroid tests administered during pregnancy reflect all this special activity. A straight T_4 estimation shows an increase, but this is deceptive—the concentration of free, ready-to-use T_4 and T_3 is only marginally increased, usually remaining within the normal range. The difference is in the "bound" form of thyroxine. Before it is released locally to do its work, thyroxine is attached to a particular protein, which carries it around in the circulatory system for when it is needed somewhere, rather like a milkman carrying quart bottles through the streets and dropping them off where they are wanted. This is the form of thyroxine that increases during pregnancy.

Nourishment

During the first three months of pregnancy your body can easily supply most of what the fetus needs. In the later months, your intake of food may fall short of requirements—not in total calories, but rather in certain nutrients, for instance calcium and various vitamins. Supplements are usually necessary.

With all the metabolic activity going on during pregnancy, it is hardly surprising that the thyroid—a major controller of metabolic processes, and kept especially busy during pregnancy—should get bigger, like a well-exercised muscle. It may not only be the extra demands on the thyroid that cause it to work so hard; the gland may also be struggling to make the best of a relative shortage of its raw material, iodine. You may live in an area where the ordinary diet provides quite sufficient iodine for you, but not for anything extra like pregnancy. It is significant that in Scotland, 80 percent of mothers-to-be develop a pregnancy goiter, while in the United States, where the dietary intake of iodine is four times greater, this is a rarity. An added drain on iodine supplies during pregnancy is an increased loss of iodine in the urine, due to the kidneys being more active than usual.

If your normal diet is near the borderline of a satisfactory iodine content, as is the case in many parts of Europe, it is wise to make sure you obtain an adequate amount from the beginning of pregnancy. This is a very small quantity, easily provided by eating seafood once or twice a week (sardines, for example, which are also an excellent source of iron and calcium), or by using iodized salt for cooking and at the table. An overload of iodine is definitely harmful to the fetus, however, so don't be too enthusiastic.

In this section we have discussed what happens during pregnancy when the thyroid is functioning absolutely perfectly. Special care is needed if the thyroid is enlarged, underactive, or overactive. These matters are addressed in the next three sections.

GOITER

If you have a simple goiter, without any symptoms of over- or underactivity, you should undergo a thyroid test—if possible one that includes an antibody screen. If your T_4 and T_3 levels are normal but the presence of antithyroid antibodies in your blood indicates an autoimmune process going on quietly (for instance, Hashimoto's disorder; see Chapter 3), you needn't take any action apart from having your thyroid checked once or twice during the pregnancy and—most importantly—afterwards.

Immunity reactions, including Hashimoto's disease, all subside during pregnancy so that the mother's system doesn't react against the baby, an "invader" in her body who is 50 percent different from her.

UNDERACTIVE THYROID

If tests indicate an underactive thyroid, whether or not you experience the slowing-down symptoms, it is essential to start thyroxine treatment right away. In this case, or if you are already on T4 for Hashimoto's disease, it is important to maintain the same dose throughout pregnancy, regardless of the results of your simple T4 tests. Recall from the disucssion earlier in this chapter that T4 levels will show an increase during pregnancy, but these results don't indicate increased levels of free thyroxine, which is what matters. If you feel hot and your pulse is fast and strong, don't assume this means you are taking too much of the hormone; pregnancy itself leads to these effects. Check with your doctor. A thyroid test—the one used to check levels of TSH (thyroid-stimulating hormone)—will indicate if you need to change your thyroxine dosage. Your baby's development depends upon a sufficient supply of thyroid hormone (see Chapter 6).

A tendency to underactive thyroid will cause problems with giving birth. Women with hypothyroid conditions feel slow, sluggish, and weak both mentally and physically, especially under the strain of childbirth.

OVERACTIVE THYROID

It is unusual for a woman to conceive if she has an unrecognized overactive thyroid, but pregnancy usually happens easily—all other factors being ideal—once she has been treated for it. Ideally, if a woman knows in advance that she is hyperthyroid and wants to plan ahead, she will get the thyroid problem resolved permanently before starting a family.

A lasting cure means either radioactive iodine or surgery. Most people, given a free choice, would prefer the medication to surgery, but a four- or five-month waiting period must elapse between taking the radioactive material and conception. After that, there is no risk to the baby's normal development. If your plans don't allow for this delay, then an operation to remove seven-eighths of the gland is a once-and-for-all option. Otherwise, you can, with care, use one of the antithyroid drugs—carbimazole, methimazole, or propylthiouracil—to control the thyroid problem while you are trying to become pregnant.

Effects on Pregnancy

If you have the common autoimmune type of overactive thyroid, your symptoms and test results will improve slightly during pregnancy because of the effect of pregnancy on the immune system. You will probably still need treatment, at least in the early stages.

Another possibility is that you develop Graves' disease for the first time when you are already pregnant. This can be difficult to recognize, because many of the indications of the overactive thyroid also crop up in pregnancy. They include feeling hot and sweaty, passing urine very frequently, a strong heartbeat, and some anxiety. Blood tests and a pulse rate that stays obstinately above ninety beats per minute, plus failure to put on weight as you should, show that your symptoms are due to illness.

Whether the overactive thyroid is a new development or already established, you must undergo treatment, for your own health and comfort and to lessen the risk of miscarriage, especially in the first few months. Unfortunately the antithyroid drugs pass through the placenta and reach the fetus. Too much of these drugs could damage the baby's thyroid. This means you must take only the smallest dose possible that still allows you to feel well. The medication usually prescribed in the United States is propylthiouracil, which is also the least harmful during breast-feeding. In Europe, carbimazole is favored during the pregnancy, with propylthiouracil after the birth.

Either way, no antithyroid drugs should be taken during the last four to six weeks before the expected due date. This is the period of maximum brain development for the baby, and it is important that the baby's own thyroid not be pushed into underactivity by the mother's antithyroid medicine. The only exception is if the doctor has some reason to think that the baby itself is at risk of being born with an overactive thyroid. There is a blood test, not available everywhere, for a specific antithyroid antibody, TRAb, which triggers Graves' disease. If TRAb is present in your blood, there is a small chance—one in seventy—of the baby's thyroid being affected. In this situation, and if there are other indications of hyperthyroidism, for instance in the fetal heart rate, it may be considered best for you to take antithyroid medication throughout the pregnancy (see Chapter 6).

It is more likely that your doctor will try to keep the antithyroid medication to a minimum. Regular testing will help to establish the dosage you need. Another option, if you have unpleasant symptoms of overactivity, is adding a beta-blocker (see Chapter 11). This will not affect the baby.

Iodine is often used to quickly slow down an overactive thyroid, but pregnant mothers cannot take any iodine-containing medicine, including wound disinfectant. Iodine can cause a large goiter to develop in the fetus if it receives a substantial dose through the mother. Radioactive iodine treatment is also out of the question, but an operation is a possibility if the overactive thyroid is causing the mother distress. The second trimester is the safest time for thyroid surgery, with the least danger of bringing on a miscarriage. Taking iodine to quiet down the gland in preparation for surgery, as described in Chapter 4, is risky to the fetus, but a combination of antithyroid medication and a beta-blocker may be used instead. Operating without settling the thyroid first can be dangerous.

Thyroid Storm

Thyroid storm is sudden, extreme overactivity of a thyroid that has run out of control. It is very rare, but creates an emergency when it occurs. It requires instant hospitalization and energetic antithyroid measures. These are life-saving and take priority over everything else.

Eclampsia—a complication of late pregnancy involving raised blood pressure—plus the birth itself can precipitate a thyroid storm if the mother's overactive thyroid has not been treated effectively. The way to prevent any risk is to meticulously keep all prenatal appointments with your doctor and to make sure you have regular thyroid tests.

Birth

Apart from the exceptional rarity of thyroid storm, giving birth will not be affected by an overactive thyroid. At the end of pregnancy the common autoimmune type of overactive thyroid is usually in abeyance, but is likely to return later.

AFTER THE BIRTH (POSTPARTUM)

Testing the Baby's Thyroid

However normal your thyroid and the pregnancy, and however beautiful your baby, it is important for him or her to have a blood test at two to five days old. This is to catch the one in four thousand chance of thyroid-hormone deficiency. Even at this low rate of incidence, thyroid-hormone deficiency is six times more likely than PKU (phenylketonuria), the other rare congenital disorder that can seriously hold back mental development if it is not spotted early. Your baby may undergo extra tests if you have had any thyroid problems (see Chapter 6).

Taking Care of Yourself

It is natural and understandable to feel exhausted but excited after the exertion of giving birth or the drama of a cesarean section. Postpartum depression affects many mothers to some extent in the first week or two after giving birth. It amounts to a few days' weepiness, although underneath you know there is everything to be happy about. In the ordinary course of things, thyroxine output dips briefly after the birth, but the effect isn't noticeable. Postpartum depression is more likely when there are antithyroid antibodies in the blood. Sometimes it seems to be the thyroxine level that is at fault, sometimes a quirk in the immune system.

Ordinarily the mother's physical and emotional strength pick up during the first month after birth, but there's a 5 percent chance of her developing either hypothyroidism or hyperthyroidism, and either condition may be associated with depression. This amounts to two hundred thousand of the four million women in the United States who become pregnant each year. The proportion who develop a thyroid disorder jumps from 5 percent to 25 percent if the woman shows signs of any other autoimmune condition. A wise precaution is to check for antithyroid antibodies early in the pregnancy and to monitor the situation particularly carefully if they are found.

Postpartum Hypothyroidism

You can suspect that your thyroid has slipped into underactivity if you become tired, weak, and depressed after you should have gotten over the initial reaction to having a baby. You find you can't concentrate, and your memory is spotty. You haven't much appetite, but your weight seems to be stuck where it was when you had the baby, instead of reverting to its prepregnancy state. This is not a severe case of the blues, or a matter of being neurotic, but a real chemical deficiency of thyroid hormones that can be demonstrated by blood tests.

In such a case it is usually worthwhile to undergo a short course of hormone replacement therapy. In three-quarters of affected women the problem is short-lived, lasting only a few months. That leaves a quarter who continue to run low on thyroid hormones indefinitely. Such a condition is all the more likely if a woman has a goiter, was previously hypothyroid, or simply has antithyroid antibodies according to the tests. If you were on thyroxine tablets before and during the pregnancy, you will certainly need to continue taking them, since the beneficial effects of pregnancy on your immune system end with the birth.

In any case, you should continue taking the medication as long as tests indicate that you need it. At the proper dosage, the tablets have no side effects and do not affect the baby if you breast-feed.

Postpartum Thyroiditis

Postpartum thyroiditis arises more often than postpartum underactivity, particularly in North America and Japan. It is an autoimmune problem, but it is not caused by the same antibodies as Graves' disease. It is also called *silent thyroiditis* because although it involves inflammation of the gland, it isn't painful or tender, unlike in de Quervain's thyroiditis.

Affected women develop the tremor, palpitations, sharp loss of weight, and general restless anxiety that are characteristic of an overactive thyroid. The patient feels hot and tired, and just when she needs all the sleep she can get, she sleeps badly. Her thyroid in most cases will remain its normal size, but it may be slightly swollen. This condition can ruin the delight of having a new baby, and sadly it is often dismissed by doctors and husbands as natural worrying and inability to cope—especially with first-time mothers.

This phase, untreated, lasts two to four months. After that a woman may shift gears into the reverse: a stage of thyroid underactivity, with slow-down, depression, constipation, and fatigue. This state of affairs can last for weeks, months, or indefinitely, or it may hardly develop at all. A goiter appears in nearly half of all those who suffer postpartum thyroiditis.

Treatment Options

If the symptoms of thyroid overactivity are mild, it may be possible to control them with a beta-blocker, which has no ill effect on breast-feeding. More likely the patient will need antithyroid medication; propylthiouracil is the drug least likely to get into the mother's milk in harmful amounts. One proviso: If your doctor wants you to have a scintigram to help confirm the diagnosis, you must stop breast-feeding for four days afterward; otherwise the radioactive iodine that is used for this special X ray might harm the baby. It is washed out of your system well before four days. (See Chapter 11 for more on scintigrams.)

If you are not breast-feeding, all options are open, including a course on steroid medicines to cut the thyroiditis short.

Future Outlook
With either underactive thyroid or postpartum thyroiditis, chances are good that the disorder will last only weeks or a few months before you are back to normal. On the other hand, if you have had postpartum thyroiditis once, you are likely to have it again when you have another child. Postpartum hypothyroidism may also recur on subsequent occasions, but the chances are somewhat less.

THYROID DISORDERS AND BIRTH DEFECTS

In January 2002, a study was presented by Drs. Adam Wolfberg and David Nagey at a meeting of the Society of Maternal-Fetal Medicine that sent a ripple of fear among women with any type of thyroid disorder who were contemplating the possibility of pregnancy in the next six to twelve months. They reported on 168 women with thyroid disease, either hypo- or hyperthyroidism, treated or untreated, who had their babies at Johns Hopkins Hospital between 1994 and 1999. A massive 18 percent of the babies had serious birth defects, such as extra fingers, cleft palate, and, most frequently, heart problems.

These results were only preliminary, and faults in the structure of the investigation need ironing out. According to the American Thyroid Association (ATA), no other studies have produced results like it, and American thyroid specialists in general have not seen higher rates of birth defects than normal among the babies of their patients. The ATA states that it "does not believe that women with well-controlled thyroid disease run a significantly higher than normal risk of having a child with a birth defect." In any event, it is prudent for mothers with thyroid disorders to work closely with their doctors before, during, and after pregnancy.

An Italian study, also published in 2002, describes additional birth defects found in newborn babies with congenital hypothyroidism. These include heart disease, nervous and eye disorders, cleft palate, and less serious abnormalities. They all crop up in the very early stages of the embryo's sojourn in the womb. The evidence suggests a strong link between congenital hypothyroidism and congenital malformation in general. As well as the genes, environmental factors play a part, and these may be modified to reduce the likelihood of thyroid problems.

French workers at Robert Debre Hospital in Paris have been following a similar line of investigation. They studied congenital abnormalities in the first-degree relatives of children with congenital hypothyroidism. They compared 241 such relatives with 217 normal controls. About 8 percent of the relatives showed abnormalities in development, affecting especially the thyroid—nine times as many as in the normal group. The implication is that congenital thyroid disorder can be inherited.

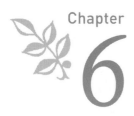

Chapter

6

Thyroid Problems in Babies Before and After Birth

IN UTERO

From the moment of conception, when sperm meets ovum and the miracle begins, your baby depends on you, the mother, for warmth, protection, nourishment, and a supply of hormones. The thyroid hormones, T_4 and T_3, have a vital role to play all the way through pregnancy and beyond. They work hand-in-hand with growth hormone for the baby's general development—including the development of such important organs as the lungs, heart, and liver—but in the following two areas their influence is dominant:

* *Brain and nervous system*, particularly the cerebral cortex, the surface layer of gray matter that covers the cerebrum (the largest part of the brain) and where ideas come from and thinking takes place; and the cerebellum, located at the lower back side of the brain, near the brain stem, and which controls the coordination of muscle movement

* *The skeletal system*, which influences height, facial features, and shape, and which includes the skull, the "strongbox" that houses the brain

In the first few weeks the fetus is almost microscopic in size, but after that there is a measurable change every week. At twelve weeks, he or she will be about four inches long, at twenty weeks about eight inches, and at forty weeks a little over twenty inches, assuming he or she has had the benefit of a normal thyroid input.

At first, the embryo absorbs all she needs directly from the tissues of the womb, where she is nestling. Everything you carry in your bloodstream, including the requisite thyroid hormones, simply soaks into the embryo. This arrangement works satisfactorily while the embryo is only a minute bundle of cells, but is inadequate by ten or eleven weeks. The fetus then needs a more efficient method. Urgently, the uterus grows, and a part of it is adapted to make the placenta. This acts as a department store for the baby's requirements, with an exclusive transport system along the umbilical cord. The placenta also acts as a kind of doorman, preventing certain substances from getting through. Although thyroid hormones are absolutely essential for fetal development, they are on the exclusion list.

While the placenta has been evolving as a supply service, the baby has been busy forming her own thyroid gland. It starts as a lump near the back of the tongue at about the third week. From there, over the ensuing weeks, the newly grown gland gradually shifts its position, moving under the jaw and into a prearranged slot in the neck. It divides into two lobes, one on each side of the voice box, joined by a narrow strip of tissue. This complicated process goes astray surprisingly seldom (see below for a discussion of some possible developmental problems in the fetal thyroid).

When the fetus is about six weeks old, the developing thyroid learns to trap iodine, and then to use it to make T_4 and T_3. By the time the fetus has to rely on the placenta for supplies from the mother, her own thyroid is capable of producing enough hormone for her needs. A small percentage still gets through from the mother's blood, but in general, from twelve weeks onward, the baby is hardly affected if the mother is hypothyroid. The baby's thyroid output increases steadily as she grows—and how she grows! It takes twenty-two weeks for the fetus to achieve a weight of one pound. The baby's weight triples to three pounds by the thirty-second week, reaches four and a half pounds at the thirty-sixth, and reaches a final weight of about seven pounds or more at forty weeks.

Building at this rate demands a high-speed metabolism—twice the rate of an adult. This is reflected in the fetus's increasing heart rate. The fetal heart can just be detected at four weeks, running at 65 beats a minute, much the same as in adults, but by the end of pregnancy the rate is more than double: 140 beats per minute. For your heart to go that fast you would have to run until you were winded. The thyroid is in charge of both metabolism and heart rate.

During the final two months of life in the womb there is a concentration on brain development, including the "governing" parts—the pituitary and the hypothalamus. These provide information and instructions to all areas of the nervous and hormonal systems, including the thyroid. At this stage and continuing through the baby's first eighteen months in the outside world, the number of brain cells increases massively. Brain cells are precious, since they cannot be produced or replaced later; they form the stock of mental material for the entire life of this new little person. A steady, sufficient flow of thyroxine is essential for this far-reaching development. No amount of money, medicine, or education can make up for a deficit of thyroid hormone before birth.

At the same time, other organs that are necessary for life, such as lungs and liver, continue developing. These are not fully mature and may not work very well when the baby is born, especially if she is premature. The same does not apply to the thyroid, unless the baby arrives extremely early, since the gland plays an important and at times life-saving role immediately after birth. The baby leaves the warmth and security of the uterus, and her supply line—the umbilical cord—is cut. The shock of the cold makes her gasp—and breathe. It also stimulates the thyroid to pour out a huge amount of T_4, and the moment the cord is cut, T_3 is also released in quantity. Although the baby's temperature plummets initially, by the time she is seven hours old it is up to normal. This is because her metabolic rate has shot up by nearly 30 percent under the influence of the extra thyroid hormones. Her metabolism peaks around the second day, running at double the adult rate. (The thyroid of a very premature infant, one younger than thirty-five weeks, cannot react so vigorously, which is one of the reasons why tiny premature babies have to start their lives in an incubator.) The hormone levels sink gradually over a few weeks, but remain higher than the adult level during the first four or five years of growth, when growth is especially rapid. In her first few days, before feeding is established, the baby must depend on her own reserves for fuel. This is in part responsible for the normal weight loss in the first week.

All of this is the everyday wonder that we take for granted, but nature isn't a production line. There are individual variations, most of them irrelevant but a few that a parent needs to watch out for in order to ward off trouble down the road for her child.

Screening tests for thyroid-hormone deficiency and for phenylketonuria are carried out when the baby is between three and five days old, once the dramatic fluctuations in thyroid activity have settled down. The method is to prick the baby's heel for a drop of blood; at this age the skin is as thin and soft in that area as it is anywhere. Screening is useful for identifying most clear cases of shortage of thyroid hormone, but no test is 100 percent accurate. The parents' careful observation provides the necessary safety net for protecting their precious baby on the threshold of its life.

A SHORTAGE OF THYROID HORMONE

Neonatal or congenital hypothyroidism occurs in about one in four thousand live births (*congenital* means existing at or dating from birth). The disastrous effects of uncorrected lack of thyroid hormone have prompted governments all over the world to set up screening programs for the newborn. Neonatal thyroid testing is required by law in all fifty states of the United States. Although there are 3,999 babies with a normal thyroid for every one with a deficiency, it is important to catch the rare newborn who would require special care all her or his life without treatment. Treatment is simple, cheap, and effective—so long as it is started within weeks of birth. From a mother's point of view, it saves her child's beauty, brains, and happiness for the rest of the child's life.

A baby's thyroid-hormone deficiency may stem from a number of sources:

- Some risks to the baby's thyroid come through his or her parents, especially the mother, and can often be avoided

- Some thyroid deficiencies result from minor developmental faults in the baby that are not life threatening but must be dealt with for full health

Problems Passed Through the Parents

Either parent may pass on genes that increase the chances of a thyroid disorder, or of an autoimmune tendency in general, but the mother is more intimately concerned, particularly if she has had a thyroid problem at any time. *If you have ever had any thyroid disorder, it is important to have your thyroid checked regularly throughout your pregnancy.*

The following are the most likely problem areas:

Recent Radioactive Iodine Treatment
Receiving treatment with radioactive iodine for overactive thyroid during pregnancy implies a major mistake in timing and/or a failure of contraceptive method. Because the delicate fetal thyroid would be destroyed, and because of the danger to the fetus of general radiation effects, a woman unlucky enough to be in this situation would probably give serious consideration to ter-

minating the pregnancy. She could try to conceive again six months after taking the radioactive iodine.

Antithyroid Medicines

Medications used to treat an overactive thyroid—such as carbimazole, methimazole, and propylthiouracil—pass through the placenta and can affect the baby's thyroid. A pregnant woman's dosage of these drugs needs careful monitoring to keep it as low as possible while still controlling her hormone levels. The antithyroid should be suspended in the last four to six weeks of pregnancy and replaced with a beta-blocker, such as propranolol, to keep her comfortable if necessary.

Antithyroid Antibodies

If you have had the autoimmune condition Hashimoto's disease at any time and you still carry a substantial amount of the antithyroid antibody in your blood, there is a small risk that the unwanted antibody will directly affect the baby's thyroid.

If you are currently on treatment for underactive thyroid from any cause, including Hashimoto's, and you are pregnant, discuss with your doctor whether you should increase your thyroxine medication slightly. In no circumstance should you reduce or stop it, even if you feel well and your thyroxine level is up.

Medicines or Foods

Certain foods or medicines the mother might ingest can upset the fetus's thyroid. Apart from a one-time dose of contrast material for an X ray of the upper digestive system (unlikely anyway during pregnancy), no harm to the baby will result unless the mother takes the risky substance consistently for some time. Medicines that matter are those containing iodides, such as some cough mixtures, as well as amiodarone for the heart; lithium, for mood illnesses; antipyrine, for asthma; sulfonamides, for infections; and some antidiabetic drugs. Discuss the matter with your doctor if you are on any of these.

On the food front, avoid an excess of the cabbage family of vegetables (brassicas), soy, corn, almonds, and kelp.

Even if you are not taking a medicine or eating much of a food that could interfere with the baby's thyroid, you may live in an area where there is a general shortage of iodine in the soil and water and thus in your diet, and you may fail to pass on enough iodine for your baby's needs. This is certainly the case in the Congo and in many parts of India, where there is also genetic thyroid weakness, and in pockets all over the world. All you need to do is ensure a reasonable intake of iodine for yourself during the pregnancy, but not an excess (see Chapter 10).

Faults in the Baby's Development

The transformation from a single cell to six or more pounds of living, breathing, crying humanity is a remarkable achievement. Even the development of the thyroid gland itself is a complicated affair. It is no wonder that sometimes—amazingly seldom—some details fail to go according to plan. We don't know the reasons for the following problems that do occasionally arise:

Agenesis
Agenesis means lack or failure of development of a body part. In the case of the thyroid, the term indicates that the gland has never grown past the bud stage. Therefore, it produces hardly any hormone. It is also known as *athyrosis*.

Dysgenesis
Dysgenesis means defective development. It is one step less serious than agenesis, but development remains incomplete. The thyroid gland may not have gotten as far as forming two lobes.

Agenesis and dysgenesis together account for 80 to 90 percent of babies born with a lack of thyroid hormone. Girls are affected twice as often as boys.

Dyshormonogenesis
Dyshormonogenesis is extremely rare. The baby's thyroid looks normal enough, but either it doesn't respond to the thyroid-stimulating hormone (TSH) from the pituitary, or it hasn't developed the ability to synthesize its own T_4 and T_3. These

hormones are complicated chemicals; it took the world's chemists until 1914 to produce a single crystal of thyroxine, and another quarter century to produce triiodothyronine, T_3.

Ectopic Thyroid

This term means that the gland is in the wrong place, having never completed the journey from the tongue to the front of the neck, or having overshot the mark and landed behind the breastbone. Most likely it never got started on its short journey, but rather developed as a reddish-purple lump on the tongue—a so-called *lingual thyroid*. If for any reason it becomes swollen, it can be a great nuisance, getting in the way of swallowing, crying, and even breathing. It may cause similar problems if it lands behind the breastbone, but usually these problems will occur much later in life (see Chapter 2). If the gland stops short of its proper destination, it may appear as a lump in the midline of the neck.

With any of these developmental mistakes the thyroid is unlikely to work perfectly. The baby may be born already hypothyroid, or the shortfall in hormones may not become obvious until later (see Chapter 7).

Symptoms

Before Birth

Since most thyroid-deficient babies seem perfectly normal when they are born, there isn't much likelihood that there will be anything obviously wrong before then. For one thing, in the womb, she could probably get by on the small amount of hormone leaking through the placenta. A thyroid-deficient baby is likely to be especially peaceful, with none of the energetic kicking mothers-to-be complain about. On the other hand, most babies settle for a quiet life toward the end of pregnancy; they simply haven't got room to move. An X ray would show if a hypothyroid baby's bone development was delayed. The last prebirth indication of hypothyroidism would be that she is more than two weeks overdue. Your doctor won't let this situation go on.

If there's a suspicion that the baby is lacking in thyroid, taking extra hormone yourself doesn't help in the later months of pregnancy—the placenta won't let it through. Occasionally it has been thought worthwhile to inject thyroxine into the amniotic fluid surrounding the fetus, but generally it is enough to check the situation when the baby arrives and start replacement treatment as soon as it becomes clear that it is needed.

After the Birth

Usually a hypothyroid baby looks perfect when he first emerges. His muscles may look slightly bigger than those of most babies, and to the doctor the fontanelle—the gap in the head bones where they haven't finally joined together—may seem a little large. The thyroid-screening test will show up positive if either the T_4 level is low or the TSH (thyroid-stimulating hormone) is high, depending on the test employed. Either result means that the baby needs a thyroid supplement, whatever the underlying cause of the shortage. Supplementation can be started when he is two weeks old, and it must be begun by the time he is two months.

If he, or more likely she, has been deprived of thyroid hormone for some time before birth, although he may be of average length and weight, his bones will show immaturity on an X ray. His brain will also show underdevelopment, and slow electrical waves will be indicated if he is given an EEG (electroencephalogram), a recording of brain activity picked up through the scalp.

Without any treatment, nothing obvious may happen for several years; still, irreversible damage will be affecting the baby's brain the whole time. Early signs of too little thyroid hormone are often difficult to recognize, and you should not blame yourself if you fail to notice them. The baby sleeps a lot, isn't terribly interested in feeding, is slow to put on weight, and just doesn't make normal growth progress. She never throws a temper tantrum or kicks and screams, and she's constipated. She may have a rather bulging tummy and perhaps an umbilical hernia, a small protuberance at the navel.

About a third of thyroid-deprived babies may exhibit one or more of the following symptoms:

- breathing difficulties or noisy breathing

- a hoarse cry

- a low temperature: 96.8 degrees Fahrenheit or less

- prolonged baby jaundice

- a big tongue

- floppy muscles

Whatever the situation at the beginning, later on the baby will be slow to reach the milestones for smiling, talking, and getting teeth, and later still she will be clumsy and poorly coordinated for skilled movements. None of this need happen, nor should the terrible mental retardation that could wreck the child's life. All that is needed is to start thyroid treatment by the time she is six weeks old. Even after a negative screening test, hints of thyroid-hormone deficiency, such as those listed above, should not be ignored.

Transient Hypothyroidism

It is not uncommon, especially if the baby was premature, for it to take several weeks for a new baby's thyroid to start producing enough thyroxine for his needs, a condition known as *transient hypothyroidism*. Another cause of a brief lack of T_4 is the use of an iodine-containing antiseptic during or after the birth. Iodine in quantity switches off the thyroid. Either way, a short course of thyroxine covers the situation, although it should be monitored by repeat tests.

Temporary Hypothyroidism

Temporary hypothyroidism may result if the baby's thyroid has been affected by the mother's taking an antithyroid medicine during pregnancy, or if some antithyroid antibodies of the

Hashimoto's type have reached the baby from her circulation. In these cases the effect usually wears off, but T_4 is typically given for the whole of the baby's first year, and is then discontinued after a satisfactory test result.

Long-Term Hypothyroidism

If the baby has been born with a rudimentary thyroid gland, or if for some other developmental reason the gland cannot supply sufficient hormone, he will need to take thyroxine by mouth indefinitely. At first he will take the medicine by spoon, with juice or formula, and later he will take the usual small, tasteless tablets. Babies and toddlers up to around age four have a rapid, active metabolism, so pound for pound they need a bigger dose than an adult.

> Baby Christine was good—too good, as it turned out. She slept through the night right from the start, and was generally cuddly and placid—"contented," her grandmother said. It was difficult to get her to nurse, so Jill felt there must be something wrong with her milk. The baby was just as bored by a bottle. The original screening test had been inconclusive, and a repeat test two weeks later showed that Christine was mildly hypothyroid, so thyroid treatment was begun. Jill and Tim were quite unprepared for the change. Christine cried loudly and a lot, often at night. She was always hungry, and needed changing far more frequently. She was generally restless, kicking off her covers and then getting cold. The final straw was that her scanty hair all fell out. Jill told the clinic pediatrician.
>
> If Christine had been having unmistakable diarrhea and losing weight, the doctor might have thought the dose of T_4 was too high. As it was, he merely reassured Jill that her noisy, obstreperous infant was healthy and normal. Her lost hair would soon be replaced by much better, silky-soft hair. Incidentally, the doctor told Jill that her breast-feeding was helpful, providing Christine with a small amount of thyroid hormone as well as the other benefits.

Nothing in life is perfect if you are a parent, but T_4 treatment for hypothyroid children proves gratifyingly effective if it is started in early babyhood and monitored monthly through the first year. Ninety percent of babies who receive this treatment wind up with a normal IQ. Young Christine is now fifteen and has just landed a scholarship to a prestigious boarding school.

Ectopic Thyroid

An ectopic thyroid gland may be able to produce a reasonable amount of hormone. It is usually considered best to suppress the gland's hormone-producing activity with iodine and antithyroid medicine (and incidentally to cause the oddly situated tissue to shrink), and to supply the baby with the thyroxine she needs by mouth. If the aberrant thyroid tissue doesn't shrink enough, is in the way, or looks unsightly—positioned in the middle of the neck, for instance—it can be removed surgically at a convenient time.

Thyroglossal Cyst

Sometimes a small swelling in the midline of the neck turns out to be a collection of fluid in a remnant of the pathway taken by the thyroid in its developmental journey down from the tongue area. Such cysts are of no importance at this stage, but may swell up or cause other problems later, and are best removed.

AN EXCESS OF THYROID HORMONE

Excessive thyroid hormone in infancy is one of the few conditions involving the thyroid in which the sexes are equally affected.

Before Birth

Hyperthyroidism before birth is a rare occurrence, and can only happen if a mother has Graves' disease, or has had it in the past and still has a high level of TRAb in her blood. TRAb is the abnormal antibody that overstimulates the thyroid in Graves' disease. It passes through the placenta from mother to fetus, affecting the fetal thyroid. The doctor would be on the alert for such an eventuality if tests showed that the mother had high TRAb. He or she would be tipped off if the baby was small, had a super-fast heart rate (more than 160 beats per minute), and showed early maturing of the bones in an X ray. Early skeletal maturation is not a bonus, but rather a disadvantage that could stunt the baby's growth. In particular, it is important that the bones of the skull do not close up ahead of schedule, since the brain has a lot of growing to do.

Treatment Options

Whether she needs it for herself or not, the mother will probably be given an antithyroid medicine and then, if she subsequently becomes short of thyroid hormone, T_4 tablets. A neat trick allows the placenta to let the antithyroid drugs through to calm down the baby's thyroid activity, even as it keeps out the thyroid hormone. In another fortunate natural arrangement, although the baby may have an excess of T_4, she cannot convert it into the much more powerful T_3 until after she has left the womb.

After the Birth

Too much thyroid hormone in a newborn baby is rare, and can only occur if the mother has, or has had, Graves' disease—particularly if she was unlucky enough to have significant eye problems (see Chapter 4 for more about this topic). Even so, the chance of the baby's being affected is only about one in a hundred. It is important to watch out for the possibility, however, since the condition can be dangerous without prompt treatment.

If you were taking antithyroid drugs during pregnancy, they may have a hangover effect on the baby and prevent the symptoms of excess thyroid from appearing for the first few hours or days. The indications include low birth weight, irritability, and a very fast heart rate (which will be taken by the doctor or midwife). A pediatrician will probably be able to detect a slight enlargement of the baby's thyroid and will note the warm, moist skin. Sometimes the baby's eyes look a little sore and puffy.

One small snag is that once the baby is separated from the mother, she can convert T_4 into powerful, fast-acting T_3, so if she is hyperthyroid, she is likely to get worse during the first few days. Tests for thyroid hormone are variable and unreliable at this stage, so the baby's appearance and behavior are more of a giveaway. If she is suffering from too much thyroid hormone, she will lose far more weight than the usual postbirth decrease of 5 to 10 percent. Although she seems to be dissatisfied, she is likely to be a poor feeder (though some babies react the opposite way and are excessively hungry). She may have a fever and is obviously ill.

Treatment Options

Medicines to calm the thyroid include an antithyroid, which can be given by injection to start with, iodine drops, and the beta-blocker propranolol. The baby also urgently needs plenty of fluids, including the right chemicals to keep the blood composition correct (electrolytes). If she is very hot, she will need cool sponging or a fan and a sedative to help her rest. Because her metabolism is racing, she will need adequate nourishment, and possibly extra oxygen. All these needs will be met, but meanwhile it is a worrisome and dramatic time.

Fortunately, after a week or so, the effect of the TRAb antibody from the mother's circulation wears off and is not replaced. In a month or two most such babies have recovered, and their parents can expect the fun and joy of having a healthy, normal baby. The antithyroid medicine can gradually be withdrawn.

Graves' Disease in a Baby

Sometimes, disappointingly, the symptoms of overactive thyroid start coming back after a newborn baby's antithyroid medication has been withdrawn.

That's what happened with baby Mark. Felicity, his mother, was unlucky enough to develop Graves' disease, with thyroid excess, partway through the pregnancy. Her condition settled down after a few weeks on methimazole, and she was able to stop taking the drug, as recommended, for the last month.

Little Mark was born rather on the small side at just under six pounds, and it soon became clear that he had an overactive thyroid. Everyone had been alert to the possibility, so he was started on treatment right away. All went well—his weight picked up, his bowels behaved reasonably, and he slept better. Unfortunately, within a week of reducing the antithyroid the diarrhea came back and he was fidgety and too restless to concentrate on nursing. These problems weren't due to Felicity's antibodies, long since cleared from Mark's system. He was making his own abnormal, thyroid-stimulating antibodies, and had independently developed Graves' disease. X rays showed that his bones were maturing somewhat too fast, so it was important for them and for his brain and nervous system to get him back on effective doses of antithyroid.

Much later, when he was starting nursery school, Mark was able to give up this medication, and from then on his T_4 and T_3 ran at normal levels. Despite this he has remained a difficult child—from the point of view of his impulsive behavior, not his physical health. If he has another relapse, the best treatment will be radioactive iodine, to deal with his thyroid once and for all.

Transient Thyroid Overactivity

Normally, a baby's system is flooded with thyroid hormones as soon as she is born and for some days afterwards. Sometimes the overload is enough to make her restless, sleepless, and dissatisfied; she may also have frequent bowel movements. She is not ill or feverish, and the whole situation evaporates within days. No treatment is needed; the condition is merely an exaggeration of the normal, physiological response to birth.

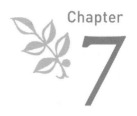

Thyroid Concerns in Children and Adolescents

Thyroid problems are uncommon in babies but quite serious when they do occur. Too little hormone can lead to irreversible long-term damage; too much can cause a life-threatening illness. In older children thyroid disorders are less of a rarity but more likely to be overlooked. It is difficult enough with an adult to recognize the onset of a thyroid problem, but at least there is a definite change in the sufferer from her usual self. Children, by nature, are changing all the time.

One of the fascinating aspects of being a parent is following how differently each child grows and develops. You don't know in advance whether he or she will be a fast or slow developer, when his growth spurt will start or her periods begin. Einstein didn't talk until he was four, while John Stuart Mill was already reading Greek at that age. My son George was small for his age and at fifteen was set on becoming a jockey. Eighteen months later he underwent a tremendous growth spurt which wrecked that plan. Girls with dreams of ballet dancing sometimes experience the same disappointment.

There are a few physical milestones early on by which a parent can informally gauge a child's growth, but these are long past by the time the majority of thyroid disorders appear in children. All in all, it is difficult for you or even the pediatrician to readily spot a possible thyroid problem. However, your child's physical, emotional, and intellectual well-being, as well as his or her happiness, can depend upon how discerning you are.

UNDERACTIVE THYROID IN CHILDREN

The ratio of girls to boys affected by underactive thyroid is two to one. Affected girls are unlikely to be younger than five; the most common age for hypothyroidism to show up in children is eight. This is because even a substandard thyroid can usually muster enough hormone for a pint-size person, but an eight-year-old uses a lot of energy and is quite big. For girls this is the threshold of puberty; the breast buds normally begin their development at this age.

It is difficult to find fault with a daughter who is slipping into thyroid deficit. She is likely to be an easy child, not given to complaining, and unlikely to be falling behind at school. If a lack of thyroid hormone emerges only after the child is older than two or three years, treatment with T_4 both ensures that her mental development will avoid permanent impairment and also possibly circumvents any noticeable slowdown.

> Clare was seven and a half when she stopped growing. It might not have been so obvious if she hadn't been a twin: Helena was unaffected. Although Clare lagged behind her sister in height, they weighed almost the same. Clare looked stocky by comparison. She had two little pads of fat just above her collarbones, but she was not fat otherwise. Her schoolwork was up to par, but her performance during PE seemed to suffer.
>
> A thyroid test showed that she was short of T_4, and a high level of the thyroid stimulator, TSH, confirmed that Clare's thyroid wasn't keeping up with the demands on it. Because the thyroid is particularly involved with the development of bone rather than the soft tissues, the latter had been less affected

when Clare's bones stopped growing. The thyroid is also essential for brain development (see Chapter 6), but that is largely completed by the end of the toddler stage. Clare was lucky that she didn't experience even a temporary fall in intelligence.

The mystery of why it had happened remained unsolved. No one in her family had a thyroid problem or even one of the other autoimmune disorders. The next step was a scintigram to show the position and amount of tissue that would take up iodine. Clare's scan revealed a small amount of iodine-containing tissue under her jaw. She had an ectopic thyroid—underdeveloped and in the wrong place. It was unable to provide enough hormone for Clare at this stage in her development.

Juvenile Hypothyroidism

Juvenile hypothyroidism is the medical term for Clare's problem. Technically it means inadequate thyroid-hormone production in a child who is past babyhood but not yet pubertal. The causes include errors in development: agenesis (also known as *athyrosis*), dysgenesis, ectopic thyroid (as in Clare's case), or the rare chemical incapacity dyshormonogenesis (see Chapter 6 for a discussion of each of these conditions). These congenital defects are slightly more likely to occur in a Down's syndrome youngster. Often they will cause problems earlier than they did in Clare's case; as discussed in the preceding chapter, if a newborn tests positive for an underactive thyroid, treatment must be started almost immediately to avoid serious problems. Less often, juvenile hypothyroidism is the beginning of Hashimoto's disease. The mitigating factor is that the outlook with juvenile hypothyroidism is far better than when thyroid-hormone deficiency affects a baby from birth.

The possible effects of juvenile hypothyroidism include the following:

» Swelling in the neck—not severe

- Slowdown of growth—especially in height

- Bones at an immature stage for the chronological age (discernible in an X ray)

- Delayed permanent teeth

- Features that look young for the child's age

- Being mildly overweight for height

- Small appetite

- Constipation

- Pale, sometimes yellow-tinged skin (maybe signalling anemia)

- Disturbed sexual development—usually delayed (no body hair, small genitals, periods delayed, poor breast development). In a minority, the opposite effect occurs, with sexual maturity coming on at eight or ten years

- Mental effects—generally slow thinking skills, poor memory, unable to concentrate, particular problems with language

No hypothyroid youngster will have all these problems; different children show the disorder in different ways. Clare, for instance, had no mental or psychological impairment. If, however, a child is increasingly slow, clumsy, inattentive, and apparently lazy, if he doesn't remember what he's told, and if he dawdles over his meals, it is easy for the parents or teacher to misinterpret the situation purely as behavioral problems. If it's hypothyroidism, talking it through or punishment won't help.

Treatment Options
A child with underactive thyroid needs thyroid tests regularly and treatment with T_4 for two years initially. Pound for pound, children need more hormone than adults, but the full dosage cannot be given at the start of treatment without a risk of se-

vere psychiatric disturbance. Because the tablets take weeks or months to make a noticeable difference, the child needs a lot of support and encouragement in the meantime. He may have a difficult time at school, so it will help if the teacher knows what's going on. The long-term results of thyroid treatment are excellent.

Muscular strength and coordination—which is required not only for sports but also to play some musical instruments—are likely to remain a little below par even after treatment. Any associated anemia, on the other hand, responds well to thyroid treatment.

The main effects of the treatment will be to make the child grow taller and more energetic. The latter change may catch parents unprepared. Sometimes treatment produces a buildup of thyroid hormones and the youngster becomes hyperactive and distractible, and may begin doing badly at school. In these circumstances the thyroid test will distinguish between successful, normal recovery and the need to reduce the medication.

The twins are both in secondary school now, but Clare is still one and a half inches shorter than Helena, and her periods started later.

Early Childhood Hypothyroidism

For the reasons discussed at the beginning of this section, hypothyroidism that develops in the very young child is less common than juvenile hypothyroidism. It is based on a congenital lack of thyroid hormone, but if the thyroid is producing a small amount of hormone, the child may be over a year old before she exhibits definite indications. These include

- sluggishness, including in bowel habits

- missing developmental milestones, including a delay in talking

- slow growth

❧ coarse, scanty hair

❧ the head seems extra large; the face becomes broader and flatter

❧ teeth are slow to appear

Testing and subsequent treatment are urgent.

"Copycat" Symptoms

Pauline's mother, Esmé, was certain in her own mind that her ten-year-old was suffering from lack of thyroid hormone. Like Esmé herself, Pauline was overweight, rather a slow child both mentally and physically. She just didn't seem to be interested in much of anything, and she also got out of PE whenever she could. The family doctor arranged thyroid tests—which all turned up negative—but allowed himself to be persuaded into trying Pauline on a short course of thyroxine. Apart from an increase in the girl's already healthy appetite, the result was zilch.

The truth of the matter was that young Pauline was depressed; she was called "Piggy" at school and got humiliatingly out of breath during sports. When she and Esmé together switched to a healthier diet, Pauline got in better shape. Her energy, concentration, and mood improved.

It is always comforting to believe that anything that goes wrong is due to "glands." It is prudent to have a thyroid test if any suspicion of a problem exists, but if the result is negative, it can only do harm to take hormone tablets. Some of the reasons why parents may suspect a thyroid disorder but be proved wrong include the following:

❧ acne

❧ delayed puberty

❧ being overweight

❧ lagging behind at school

* constipation

* being physically inactive

* a passive attitude, lack of assertiveness (especially in a
  boy)

These characteristics could figure in a hypothyroid disorder, but just as often they may merely be aspects of individual variation, plus possibly, as in Pauline's case, depression. The laboratory tests are the best guide.

OVERACTIVE THYROID IN CHILDREN

Hyperthyroidism is, as usual, more prevalent in girls, increasingly so as they grow older and produce more estrogen, the female sex hormone. When boys do have this disorder, however, they tend to suffer more severely.

It is rare for a child to have an overactive thyroid before the age of five; the usual age of onset is around ten. There is a genetic link, and thyroid problems tend to run in families. A predisposition may be triggered into unmistakable overactivity by several types of stress: emotional, as in a traumatic family breakup; an infection or some other physical trouble; or occasionally an excess of iodine. Iodine overload may come about via the milk the child drinks, and is most likely to occur in the first half of the year, when cows are eating new spring grass, which contains more iodine than their winter fodder. Whatever the cause, the stress can set off the autoimmune type of overactive thyroid, Graves' disease, in a child who is constitutionally susceptible.

The hitch is that an overactive thyroid doesn't show up in young people in the way you might expect.

Philip was nearly expelled from his prestigious prep school. His father was furious, and his mother wondered where they'd gone wrong. It all dated back to a nasty bout of streptococcal sore throat. Phil was eleven at the time, and from then on he became more and more difficult to cope with. He was fidgety and always up to something, then became dreadfully upset when he was reprimanded. He had been in the top third of his class at school, but now he was near the bottom. Even his handwriting was sloppy.

A counselor at the child-guidance clinic tried talking to Phil, to no avail. Then his mother had the idea that he might have worms. He was eating enormously but was as skinny as a rake. The pediatrician ran a battery of tests, and an excess of thyroid hormones showed up.

Symptoms

Physical Problems
In younger kids in particular:

* prolonged bed-wetting

* frequent bowel movements

  At all ages:

* neck swelling, perhaps slight, in 95 percent of cases

* poor sleep and daytime restlessness

* weight loss in 80 percent of cases

* weight gain in 20 percent of cases

* enormous appetite

* tremor

* itchy skin, with fidgetiness

* being slightly tall for the child's age

* becoming easily tired

* weak muscles

* dislike of hot weather and hot rooms

* mildly sore eyes, with puffy lids

Mildly sore eyes are fairly common in children with overactive thyroid. The condition is not serious, nor does it necessarily indicate an infection, like conjunctivitis. Treatment with artificial tears helps.

Mood and Behavior Problems

These may be so obvious and so troublesome that parents at first hardly notice anything else wrong:

- difficulties in relationships with family members, friends, and teachers

- disruptions at school—short attention span, easily distracted, unable to keep still

- easily upset, bursting into tears, throwing temper tantrums, often rude and rebellious, moody and uncooperative

Early Signs

The most readily noticed early signs of hyperthyroidism include the child developing a small goiter after going through an emotional stress. If parents promptly recognize the signs of the illness and have the condition treated right away, chances are favorable for nipping the problem in the bud and reaching a full recovery.

Treatment Options

When thyroid tests have confirmed that an overactive thyroid is at fault, a long course of treatment is in prospect. There are no quick miracles; the medication must be built up gradually, and the results are gradual too. A child in this situation needs endless patience and understanding, however difficult she may be. She is genuinely in turmoil, and doesn't know why.

Antithyroid Medicine

The first step is to get the youngster started on an antithyroid drug. Methimazole (trade name Tapazole) is preferred, since it

need only be taken once a day. A more complex routine is difficult for any child to remember, let alone a child with a restless
mind caused by excess thyroid hormone. The dosage is monitored by how the child feels and behaves, and after some months
can often be reduced without ill effect.

About one child in three develops side effects from the medication. These are not usually dangerous, but are unpleasant, for
instance, feeling sick, experiencing pain in the joints, or developing a rash. Very occasionally a more serious problem called *agranulocytosis* threatens to interfere with the production of white
blood cells. A sore throat and/or mouth ulcers signify this condition, which requires urgent medical attention.

Typically, the medicine is continued for one to two years
before trying the effect of stopping it. If the symptoms return,
the medication must be resumed for another year. The entire
time the child is on an antithyroid drug she or he must see the
doctor and have a blood test every month. This can be incon-
venient at times.

It is a good sign if any neck swelling is reduced during treatment, but if the goiter enlarges it indicates that the medication
has been too effective and has pushed the thyroid into underactivity. This calls for a reduction in the antithyroid and/or the
addition of replacement thyroxine for fine-tuning.

Radioactive Iodine

If side effects make it uncomfortable or unsafe to continue with
a particular antithyroid medication, another may be tried, but
most likely it, too, will fail to produce a lasting cure. In this case
another form of treatment must be substituted. Until ten or fifteen years ago most experts considered radioactive iodine to be
unsuitable for growing children, in case it interfered with their
development and in particular their fertility later. These fears
have been proved groundless, and radioactive iodine is becoming
the most favored treatment for children with overactive thyroid.

Since the chance of achieving satisfactory control of the disorder with antithyroid medicines is only 50 percent, some par-

ents and doctors together decide to go for radioactive iodine before trying any other treatment. Radioactive iodine is successful in 92 percent of children, usually requiring only one dose. In nearly all cases the thyroid is switched off completely, necessitating thyroxine replacement indefinitely. Unlike the case with antithyroid medications, this treatment does not require returning to the doctor for frequent checkups.

Surgery

Sometimes parents feel so apprehensive about the possible adverse effects for their child of using radioactive iodine that they prefer surgery, if antithyroid treatment proves unsatisfactory. For a few days before the operation the thyroid is settled down with iodine drops and the beta-blocker propranolol. Although surgery traditionally offers the advantage of producing an immediate cure, it is not always completely successful, especially in children. In about one-sixth of them, the effects of overactive thyroid return some time after the operation. Then the usual choice is radioactive iodine after all.

General Support

Whichever specific form of treatment is used, other, more general supportive measures are also needed:

- super-generous nutrition, rich in protein and carbohydrate

- extra calcium (found in cheese, milk, sardines)

- vitamin supplements—there may be shortages of vitamin A and the B group in particular (milk, cheese, egg yolk, and carrots are rich in vitamin A or its precursor beta-carotene; whole wheat, legumes, eggs, liver, meat, and greens provide the B group)

The excess of thyroid hormones will have induced an abnormally high metabolic rate that burns up food incredibly fast. The demand will continue for weeks after the illness itself is under control.

With so much internal as well as external activity, the child needs rest in both body and mind. A sedative may help. Don't be disappointed if it takes a long time for his or her mood and behavior to calm down. This disorder is a major test for the parents, so try to make everything else as easy for yourselves as possible. You deserve it.

THYROID CANCER

Cancer of the thyroid is uncommon at any age, and extremely so in childhood. Boys and girls are equally unlikely to be affected, but the risk is enhanced if the child has ever been exposed to X rays in the neck area. Until recently, X rays were sometimes used as a treatment for acne, thymus enlargement, recurrent tonsillitis, or chronic ear infections, but this practice has been stopped. Fortunately, thyroid cancer is a particularly mild type in children; it's also slow-growing and has a 95 percent cure rate. The basic symptom is a painless, hard lump in the neck that gradually gets bigger.

Treatment Options

Radioactive iodine is used in a dose sufficient to kill off cancer cells, including any secondary spread. It incidentally prevents the healthy thyroid tissue from making its hormones, but this is easily remedied with thyroxine tablets.

ADOLESCENTS

Adolescent Goiter

Adolescence is a period of great change and growth. There is a dramatic spurt in height and development, usually starting at about age eleven in girls and two or three years later in boys. The reproductive organs mature, and the secondary sexual characteristics appear, including breast development and the menses in girls, and facial hair and a deepening voice in boys. The shape and bony structure of the face and pelvis alter, too.

All this places huge demands on the metabolism, which must supply the materials and energy for growth. Since the rate of metabolism depends on the thyroid, the gland is called upon for extra activity. It is at this stage that a goiter commonly develops. The thyroid may swell up simply because it is so busy, or it may be struggling to make the most of a supply of iodine that was borderline before, and is now inadequate for so much growth and tissue activity. One possible result, in a susceptible youngster, may be that the stress on the gland stimulates the formation of the unwanted antibodies of Hashimoto's disease. Sixty-five percent of adolescent goiter is due to this disorder. In most cases, at least one of the parents also carries the applicable antibody, even if that parent hasn't been aware of any thyroid problems.

An adolescent goiter may slightly decrease in size over two or three years, and remain smaller unless some new stress affects the metabolism. Having a baby, an infection or physical illness, or an emotional disaster may upset the thyroid again, or a major fault in the diet may have the same effect.

Estrogen, the female sex hormone, increases the sensitivity of the thyroid to stimulus. This accounts for the great majority of girls with noticeable adolescent goiters. In the seventeenth century, the painter Sir Peter Lely made portraits of many of the beautiful and high-born ladies of the English court. Nearly all show the gentle outward curve of a small goiter in their necks.

Underactive and Overactive Thyroid

At this age, underactive and overactive thyroid problems will be due to one or the other type of autoimmune disorder: Hashimoto's or Graves' disease, respectively. The symptoms and signs may be any of those associated with either the adult or childhood versions of the disease. The moodiness and unpredictability of teenagers may be partly due to the normal increase in T_3, the more powerful of the thyroid hormones, at this stage. If the moods become extreme, parents should consider having their child's doctor check for a thyroid upset. Depression and lethargy signal too little hormone, while alternating bouts of energy and exhaustion may result from too much. Either way, affected youngsters are more than usually uncooperative and touchy.

The thyroid is closely involved in sexual development. Even a simple adolescent goiter often swells up seven to ten days before each menstrual period. At this key age any thyroid disturbance affects the sexual characteristics.

Shortage of Thyroid Hormone

Hypothyroidism usually delays the onset of puberty, but it may have the opposite effect, causing the child to become sexually mature, with all the accompanying physical characteristics, at eight or ten years old. Fortunately this precocious development regresses back to the normal stage with thyroid treatment. In young women who have already reached puberty in the ordinary way when the thyroid-hormone deficiency shows itself, the periods become heavy, irregular, and painful. Anemia is common in hypothyroidism, due to a lack of T_4, but some girls may also experience a lack of iron from excessive blood loss each month.

Excess of Thyroid Hormone

In the case of hyperthyroidism in adolescents, sexual development is likely to be delayed. The periods may fail to begin, or if they do begin, they may become scanty and gradually stop. Boys remain immature, having small organs for a longer time period than their peers, and they are not interested in sex.

> Alison was sixteen-and-a-half when she began losing weight—far more successfully, it seemed, than the other girls at school who were into dieting. She was pleased. Her periods stopped, and she seemed to lose all her feeling for her friends. However cold it was, she would wear only the thinnest, skimpiest garments. The doctor considered several possibilities applicable to Alison's age group.

The weight loss, the lightening and loss of her periods, her awkwardness with her friends, and her insensitivity to the cold could all add up to an overactive thyroid. On the other hand, her pleasure at losing weight and the complete absence of periods would fit in with a diagnosis of anorexia nervosa. A thyroid test showed a high level of thyroid hormones in her blood; they would have been abnormally low in anorexia.

Anorexia Nervosa

This so-called dieters' disease is most likely to affect girls between fourteen and eighteen. The key symptoms are the following:

- serious weight loss

- cessation of periods

- refusal to eat enough to maintain a normal weight (or in some cases deliberate vomiting to get rid of food)

The thyroid reacts to starvation by reducing its output of T_4 and converting it into inactive reverse-T_3 (rT_3). This slows the metabolism, the rate at which food is used up. The heart rate slows and, because of the poor circulation, the individual's hands and feet are cold and blue. Her skin is parched, her hair is dry, and she feels deadly cold—but she's happy to be losing weight. She withdraws from her friends and has near tantrums if anyone tries to make her eat. The cause, and the cure, are psychological. She also needs a carbohydrate-based, nourishing diet. The thyroid responds rapidly to carbohydrate.

Drastic Slimming, with the Use of Amphetamines or Other Pills

This dangerous habit typically affects older adolescent girls. One risk is that if there is an autoimmune tendency in the family, the individual may be precipitated into Graves' disease, characterized by a high level of thyroid hormones. Some diet pills contain thyroxine, which has a direct thyrotoxic effect. The treatment involves eliminating the use of diet pills, taking plenty of nourishment—especially protein and carbohydrate—and controlling such symptoms as tremor or palpitations with a beta-blocker for the time being. Further thyroid testing is required to assess the situation in a few weeks.

Substance Abuse

Ecstasy, crack, speed, acid, and heroin can cause weight loss, tremor, nervousness, and disruption of the menstrual cycle. These signs can arouse suspicions of an overactive thyroid, but tests show a normal or reduced level of the hormones.

Emotional Stress

At this sensitive, insecure age, despite whatever front they put on, adolescents are greatly affected by emotional upsets. Weight loss, frequent bowel movements and urination, rapid pulse, sweating, tremor, poor sleep, restlessness, disrupted periods, and tearfulness all may have a psychological basis, even though the symptoms match those of overactive thyroid. Blood tests will indicate whether or not the origins of the problems lie with the thyroid. If the gland is exonerated, psychiatric help is then needed, often involving the parents.

Anorexia nervosa and drastic dieting with the aid of chemicals are mostly girls' problems. Drugs and emotional stress can affect either sex. For adolescents especially, psychiatric or psychological counselling and support are important when something goes wrong, whether it is a thyroid disorder or some other problem. Other treatments can run concurrently. Alison took carbimazole for a year, but she still sees her therapist from time to time. She is well and happy in high school.

Chapter 8

Thyroid Issues in Women over Fifty

Thyroid problems are relatively common from age fifty onward. Awareness of them is enormously important because of the mental misery and dangers to physical health they can cause. Yet they frequently go unrecognized and untreated.

The trouble is that in this age group thyroid disorders don't present themselves in the well-defined fashion that they do in younger adults. The symptoms that do appear can be easily explained away as something quite different—as a result, for instance, of menopause, diabetes, high blood pressure, or depression. Worst of all, sufferers may endure them without complaint due to a belief that they're caused simply by age—"the sort of thing I should expect at this age." When a patient doesn't complain about her malaise, the doctor won't know there is anything wrong, and thus cannot undertake the investigations that might reveal a totally curable thyroid problem.

Just as all babies are screened for thyroid abnormalities, so those of us who are middle-aged and older should have a routine thyroid check, without waiting for evidence of disease to force the issue.

Typically, the basic metabolic rate (BMR) slows down gradually over the years; this is because middle-agers are on a maintenance rather than a building program. The amount of T_4 in the bloodstream remains much the same, but since less is used up, less needs to be produced. The turnover—the time it takes to replace the body's stock of thyroxine—increases from seven to nine days. There is also proportionately less need for the super-active hormone T_3, so slightly less T_4 is converted to T_3. There is measurably less T_3 in circulation after age eighty-five.

This mild metabolic scaling back occurs partly because we don't usually participate in as much energetic physical activity as we did earlier, so there is less reason to burn fuel fast. Even when we are resting, the metabolic rate is more leisurely—as an economy measure and also to reduce strain on the heart and the breathing apparatus.

This doesn't mean we should accept feeling dull and lethargic or less mobile than before, but the slower metabolism does reduce the speed with which we can gear up to meet a sudden demand on muscular energy. It also makes us more vulnerable to cold. This can be an annoyance to the naturally frugal, whose instinct is to be economical with the heating.

> Judy's husband, Dick, was like that: an avid turner-off of switches. Usually Judy managed unobtrusively to switch them on again, but things reached a crisis point when Dick retired and Judy developed an underactive thyroid. Neither of them realized what was happening, although for some time Judy had noticed that her fingers turned dead white whenever there was a chill in the air. Gradually she felt less and less like making any effort to keep the house warm, or indeed like doing anything at all. Dick took on a lot of the energetic chores and did not notice the temperature.
>
> During a cold snap one day, returning home from a trip to the supermarket, Dick found the house icy and Judy slumped in a chair, barely conscious. She was slipping into a myxedematous coma and hypothermia. She recovered in the hospital,

where her thyroid-hormone deficiency was discovered. Now that Judy is established on her T_4 supplement she is alert to the situation and keeps the house warm.

MEDICINES THAT MAY AFFECT THYROID TESTS

One of the features of getting into your second half-century is an increased likelihood of being on some kind of regular medication. Some medicines actually affect thyroid function directly, while others merely distort the test results.

High T_4 Reading
A high T_4 reading may be caused by the following:

- too high a dose of thyroxine

- iodides in medication—for instance, cough mixtures, amiodarone (for the heart; men are especially affected), or disinfectant for wounds and sores

- estrogens—for hormone replacement therapy or prostate problems, or in the contraceptive pill (less likely to be a source at this age)

- levodopa or bromocriptine—for Parkinson's disease

- kelp—a seaweed-based health food

- thiazide diuretics—these produce only an apparent increase in T_4, due to a loss of fluid that makes the blood more concentrated

Low T_4 Reading
A low T_4 reading may be caused by the following:

- iodides in medication and food (including amiodarone and kelp; see above), which sometimes switch off T_4 production instead of stimulating it

- antiepileptic drugs such as carbamazepine

- diazepam (Valium)

- chlorpromazine, a major tranquillizer

- androgens and body-building steroids

- some medicines for arthritis and rheumatism

- salicylates, including aspirin

- co-trimoxazole, an antibacterial drug

- chlorpropamide and other antidiabetic drugs

- heparin, to prevent clotting

Reduced Conversion of T_4 to T_3

T_3 readings may be reduced and T_4 may go up slightly due to the effects of beta-blockers such as propranolol, nadolol, and stanozolol.

In the over-fifties age group, test results are much more subject to day-to-day variation, whether or not any medicine is being taken. Repeat thyroid tests may be necessary to check inconsistent readings (see also Chapter 11).

UNDERACTIVE THYROID

Hypothyroidism is increasingly prevalent in people fifty and over, and it is fourteen times as likely in a woman as a man. The chances of developing it are around 5 percent per year if the individual carries the antithyroid antibodies in her blood—and nearly one in five people do, without ever having had any thyroid problems. Some people become hypothyroid as the end result of treatment with radioactive iodine or surgery for Graves' disease, even if the treatment was years earlier. For others it may be the effect of one of the medicines mentioned above. For the majority it will mean a late, slow development of Hashimoto's disease—a reaction to abnormal antibodies.

Symptoms

It is important not to ignore any pointers to hypothyroidism for fear of being a nuisance or of making a fuss about nothing. Of course, other reasons may exist for the complaints you have, but if it is a thyroid problem it needs treatment.

Physical Symptoms
These may include the following:

Slowing down   Everything takes twice as long.

Constipation   This is never due to age alone, but can be brought on by too little exercise, failure to drink enough fluids, and certain medicines such as cold remedies and antidepressants—or it can be caused by too little thyroid hormone.

Loss of weight   This is in contrast to the weight gain that is typical of underactive thyroid at other ages. Appetite is reduced as well.

Rapidly aging facial appearance   The face is also sallow and puffy, without its normal expressiveness. This happens over a matter of months. Other people are likely to notice it in the patient, and to worry.

Thinner and finer hair   Instead of going gray, the hair tends toward a dull, darkish hue. Oddly, hypothyroid patients may also lose the outer third of each eyebrow.

Raynaud's disease   As happened with Judy (see pages 128–129), the fingers may go dead and pale even in the slight cold. They recover painfully when they are warmed up.

Hearing loss   The individual may become increasingly hard of hearing, and may also suffer from vertigo and the constant ringing in the ears called tinnitus. It is all due to thyroid-hormone deprivation, which affects the hearing and balance nerves.

Hoarse voice   Friends will be more aware of this than you. The problem isn't due to the normal effects of maturity.

High blood cholesterol   This can lead to angina (chest pain triggered by exercise), fainting, convulsions, and shortness of breath. Typically, the thyroid hormones work to keep the cholesterol in circulation at a lower level.

Anemia   Anemia can be caused by lack of thyroxine, and it compounds the problem of clogged arteries by reducing the quality of the blood that does get through.

Heart problems   These are the most likely reason why a person over age fifty might consult her doctor if she has an underactive thyroid. The rhythm of the heartbeat may be disturbed, which makes the heart pump inefficiently. This in turn leads to congestion in the body, with swelling ankles and shortness of breath. Anginal chest pain can increase, occurring even during rest, and the blood pressure may increase slightly. The start of treatment may make matters worse. The heart may have been able to cope with the slowed-down metabolism and heart rate of too little thyroid hormone, but it is put under strain when there is an overall speeding up. The answer is a two-pronged treatment: thyroxine, which is necessary to rescue general health from deterioration, and propranolol or digoxin to protect the heart from overworking.

Rheumatic problems   Most common are muscular weakness and "rheumaticky" aching, especially in the neck. Although the muscles don't look smaller, and may even be slightly bigger, there is a loss of active, working muscle cells, made up for in bulk with connective tissue, collagen, and fibrous tissue, which serves as a sort of packing material. Arthritis that causes muscle pain may affect the small joints, but lack of thyroxine seldom involves knees and hips. Gout, rheumatoid arthritis, and polymyalgia rheumatica are all more likely in sufferers of the Hashimoto's autoimmune type of thyroid underactivity. So is carpal tunnel syndrome, which is recognized by the sensation of pins and needles in the hands (see Chapter 3).

Goiter   This is not likely to be a feature in the fifty-plus age group, and any long-standing swelling will probably have shrunk, if anything.

Mental and Emotional Symptoms

The symptoms that show themselves in your mood, personality, and mental speed and efficiency are often the most distressing to endure. Added to this, other people tend to regard these symptoms with impatience, rather than offering the help and sympathy that physical disorders attract. Psychological changes may also be not only the worst but also the first to appear.

If these symptoms affect you, you find yourself inexplicably less alert and confident. You have lost all interest and enthusiasm in your favorite activities. You can't seem to care about the people who mean most to you. You may feel pointlessly agitated, hopelessly indecisive, or just empty. Your memory and concentration are apt to be erratic, and you can't deal with the sort of problems you would have sailed through before. You sleep for a long time and may drop off during the day, but you never feel refreshed. This is because you are missing out on stage-4 sleep, the deepest and most reviving sleep.

All this could indicate a severe depressive illness, or your relatives may wonder if you have Alzheimer's disease. If the problem is an underactive thyroid, antidepressants will be useless and will make any constipation worse, but thyroid tests will be positive. This is the signal to start thyroxine treatment gently.

Since the shortage of thyroid will have built up over many months, during the recovery period you will seem miraculously to grow younger. You will be livelier, happier, and more mobile week by week. Your feelings of affection will come out of the deep freeze, as will your ability to think and work things out.

You will have to remain on the tablets indefinitely, but this is a small price to pay for regaining your true self. At your age the dosage need not be large, but without it you would be at risk of degenerating into an immobile, brainless lump.

Since the treatment of underactive thyroid is so simple and magically effective, it would be a tragedy not to take it. If you are developing the disorder, you may exhibit several or only one of the symptoms that point to its possibility. If there's any question, the sensible move is to go to your doctor for a checkup. You've nothing to lose, and much to gain.

Myxedema

Myxedema is the ultimate stage in underactive thyroid; it is named after the typical puffiness (edema) of the skin that accompanies the other signs and symptoms of thyroid deficiency. There are likely also to be problems in the nervous system in particular, including the sensation of pins and needles anywhere in the body. Unsteadiness, with a real risk of falling, results from thyroid-hormone deficiency in the cerebellum, the part of the brain that coordinates movement. Myxedema is unlikely in the younger age groups.

Myxedema Coma

Myxedema coma is a dangerous slide into unconcsciousness that most often affects elderly women—seventy-five-plus—who live alone. The final trigger that brings it on is often another illness, such as a bladder infection or chest infection. Alcohol, sedatives, or such major tranquillizers as chlorpromazine (Thorazine) increase the risk, as does neglect of nourishment, warmth, and comfort. The body temperature may fall too low for an ordinary clinical thermometer to register it.

This is where Judy (see page 128–129) was heading. She was lucky her husband came home when he did, since even today this development carries a high mortality. As recently as the early 1960s only one in five victims of myxedema coma recovered.

The treatment consists of gradual rewarming with blankets in a room of normal temperature, urgent T_4 or T_3 by injection or via a tube to the stomach, antibiotics, and sometimes steroids temporarily.

Myxedema Madness

With myxedema, chances are that a friend or relative, rather than the sufferer herself, will notice something dreadfully wrong. This is particularly true of the serious psychiatric illness that can be part of the condition. Whereas it's typical for the hypothyroid patient to feel profoundly lethargic and depressed, if the condition has progressed to this stage she may become irrational or even delirious. More likely, she feels persecuted, suspecting plots and deadly threats from neighbors, acquaintances, television, or the government. Reason and resassurances are useless; psychiatric help is essential, preferably in a hospital where the whole illness can be brought under control.

OVERACTIVE THYROID

The chances of having an overactive thyroid increase with age: Ten percent of all cases crop up in the over-seventies age group. Around eight times as many women as men are affected. In fact, 2 percent of women ages sixty and over are known to be suffering from too much thyroid hormone, and this doesn't count those who remain undiagnosed. How many of your thin, agitated, and inefficient middle-aged acquaintances might be struggling with an overload of T_4?

Four out of five individuals whose thyroids become overactive at this age are harboring the peculiar thyroid-stmulating antibodies of Graves' disease. At least half of them have no detectable goiter; a few have a smooth, allover swelling; and the rest have a long-standing, knobby, multinodular goiter that has started acting up, perhaps in only one nodule. Other, less common causes include the early phase of de Quervain's inflammation of the thyroid (see Chapter 2), hashitoxicosis (see Chapter 4), or the effects of medication (see Chapter 10). Men are especially vulnerable to a reaction with amiodarone. Trouble from this useful drug cannot be dealt with simply by stopping it, since it lurks in the system for months. Beta-blockers are the first line of defense, while a strategy for both heart and thyroid is worked out.

Symptoms

Just as with too little thyroid hormone, too much produces very different effects after age fifty compared to earlier ages.

Heart Disorder

This is the major set of symptoms, often the first to appear, and vitally important. It shows up in the following:

* palpitations

* rapid, irregular pulse (atrial fibrallation)

* tight, choking chest pain with exertion (angina)

* breathlessness with the slightest effort

* swollen ankles

* a purplish complexion at times

* exhaustion

* fainting spells

* raised blood pressure

The giveaway feature is a disappointing lack of improvement in the symptoms with the usual heart drugs, unless the excess thyroid is also corrected.

Apathetic Thyrotoxicosis

Among those of us over fifty, a sizeable minority reacts to too much thyroid with symptoms that are the oppsite of the usual ones. The term for this state of affairs is *apathetic* or *masked thyrotoxicosis*.

Regular Hyperthyroidism	Apathetic Hyperthyroidism
Peak age forty-plus	Peak age sixty-seven
Big appetite	No appetite; nausea
Frequent bowel movements	Constipation
Anxiety	Depression, apathy
Restlessness	Lethargy
Comes on over months	Takes several years

Other Symptoms

In both regular and apathetic thyrotoxicosis, watch for the following symptoms:

- severe weight loss (of between ten and thirty pounds)

- worsening of asthma or other breathing problems

- warm skin (but not sweaty at this age)

- fatigue

- uneasy, unrefreshing sleep

- extreme weakness in the big muscles, with pain and stiffness

- "frozen shoulder" from inflammation of the covering of the joint

- thinning of the bones, with a risk of fracture

Occasionally you may also come across the following symptoms:

- prominent eyes (this problem is less likely at this age, and it can be caused by a disease of the major airways— the trachea and bronchi—rather than the thyroid)

❧ thickening and purplish-red discoloration of the skin over the shins

Treatment Options

The first essential is to pinpoint what precisely is at fault using the standard blood tests for thyroid hormones, possibly a scintigram, and, in the case of a single nodule, a fine-needle aspiration (see Chapter 11 for descriptions of these tests). If you have heart symptoms, you may need a beta-blocker or digoxin or both, in addition to the treatment for overactive thyroid. Radioactive iodine is the preferred treatment for overactive throid, with surgery second, since in middle age there is more risk of side effects with protracted use of antithyroid drugs such as carbimazole.

The thyroid, like other parts of the body, needs to be treated with consideration at this age. That means undergoing a short course of a beta-blocker, combined with an antithyroid if necessary, to calm the overactivity before undertaking either of the two major treatments.

If you have a long-standing goiter, it is essential to undergo one of the permanent, curative processes, but if you have Graves' autoimmune disorder, with no noticeable goiter or only a small, smooth swelling, there's a slight chance that the disorder will die down with a short course of antithyroid and will not relapse.

Laura and Elspeth are sisters, not very much alike and with five years between them. At the time all the problems started, each was worried about the other. Laura, the elder, looked dreadful. She had lost so much weight that her clothes hung on her as though she were a coat hanger, and in spite of pressure from her husband and her sister, she picked at her food and ate next to nothing. Laura herself was worried, but she wouldn't go to the physician because she was afraid of what she might be told. She'd read somewhere that between the ages of sixty and seventy was the cancer decade, and everyone knows that you lose weight with cancer. Anyway, she felt too tired to bother.

It was only when the doctor came to check on Laura's eighty-five-year-old mother that he noticed Laura's thinness and her agitated manner. He insisted, in the kindest way, on giving her a complete workup at his office. Her overactive thyroid came to light, and she was soon on the road to recovery.

Elspeth also had a thyroid problem. She'd had a goiter for years, but it didn't give her any trouble so she ignored it. She'd always been overweight and thus tried to eat sensibly, but she now seemed to feel hungry all the time. This wasn't why she went to the doctor; the problems bothering her were constant fatigue, shortness of breath, and swollen ankles. The doctor listened to Elspeth's heart and did an electrocardiogram. Together with her fast, irregular heartbeat, the electrical recording showed that she had atrial fibrillation. This, along with her being overweight, would certainly account for her symptoms, but the goiter and the fact that there were thyroid problems in Elspeth's family reminded the doctor to ask some more questions, and to send Elspeth off for a blood test. The physician was interested to hear that Elspeth had recently begun suffering from waves of anxiety that had been coming on for no reason.

The test results showed that Elspeth, like Laura, had an excess of thyroid hormone, although the effects on the two sisters were quite different. Because of Elspeth's heart condition, the doctor was particularly careful to reduce the heart strain and the excess T_4 gradually, before giving her radioactive iodine. If the goiter had been awkwardly big, or if there had been a single, particularly large nodule, the choice for treatment would have veered toward surgery.

Both sisters now have to take thyroxine daily, ever since a few months after radioactive iodine treatment, but this is a small inconvenience for keeping in good health.

CANCER

From age fifty on, anyone who finds a lump in their neck or anywhere else thinks of cancer. Even if there isn't anything new except an increase in size of part of a goiter you've had for years, it needs to be addressed. The least worrisome kind is the general lumpiness of an established multinodular goiter.

If there is a tumor, a scintigram will highlight it and will give an indication of its type; several varieties of thyroid tumor exist. Fine-needle aspiration, followed by biopsy, is especially useful for checking out a single suspicious nodule. (See Chapter 11 for details of both these techniques.) For the best results, it is important to find out what's going on and start whatever treatment is appropriate without delay.

Between ages sixty and eighty the risk of a thyroid cancer is 3½ in 100,000; it decreases after eighty. Most thyroid cancers are very slow-growing, and often a thyroid cancer is discovered only after the person has died of something else. Apart from an enlarging lump, the only symptoms, if any, may be hoarseness without a sore throat and, very rarely, some discomfort in swallowing.

Treatment

Some types of thyroid cancer are best treated by an operation followed by radioactive iodine, but radioactive iodine alone is usually all that is necessary. A sizeable dose is used, which knocks out the good as well as the bad thyroid cells, so the patient must take thyroxine forever afterward. The results are excellent.

OTHER ILLNESSES

It is more likely after age fifty than earlier in life that a woman's body will have acquired some signs of wear and tear. These may have no relation to her thyroid, but they need care in their own right. They may also cause symptoms that she might think are due to thyroid problems. For instance, it is commonplace to develop diabetes in middle age, and this can cause lassitude that might be mistaken for a thyroid disorder. Likewise, coronary or rheumatic heart disease can develop with a perfect thyroid, as can arthritis of any type, bronchitis, and emphysema.

While the thyroid can be upset temporarily by an acute illness such as flu or shingles, it will right itself automatically once the sickness is past. Even long-lasting problems are only likely to throw the thyroid temporarily out of kilter due to the medicines a patient may have to take (see Chapter 10 for a discussion of these medications and their possible effects). The good thing about a thyroid problem is that it can nearly always be put right and leaves no lasting damage.

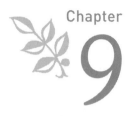

The Other Thyroid Hormone

Most of us think of the thyroid hormones as T_4 and T_3, which control our metabolism. But they are not the whole story. About thirty years ago, another thyroid hormone, calcitonin, was discovered. It is made in the thyroid gland by some special cells—the "C" cells. Calcitonin is also produced by the parathyroid and thymus glands.

Calcitonin affects the way the body deals with calcium, the important mineral in bones and teeth. Calcium is also vital for the working of the automatic muscles—for instance, those in the bowels, the bladder, and the heart. Too much or too little calcium in the blood can literally be fatal. The bones are used as a handy, on-the-spot repository for excess calcium, and the kidneys wash out any surplus via the urine.

The calcium level is largely controlled by the parathyroid glands, four little chunks of tissue attached to the back of the thyroid lobes. To do this, they produce their own special hormone, parathyroid hormone (PTH), but they are relatively slow to react to changes in the amount of calcium in circulation, taking three or four hours to do so. This is where calcitonin steps in. The thyroid's "C" cells respond within minutes if the calcium level goes up by 10 percent. They can rev up calcitonin production to six times the normal.

This process typically comes into action after a meal, especially one including plenty of calcium (from cheese, milk, yogurt, or sardines, for example). Under the influence of the surge of calcitonin, appetite is switched off almost immediatley and the blood is cleared of excess calcium by dumping the surplus into the bones. Within an hour, and continuing for several days, extra bone-building cells are produced to organize the extra calcium, but in the longer term, calcitonin slows down bone turnover.

PAGET'S DISEASE

Bones, like other tissues, are constantly being replaced and renewed. In Paget's disease, which affects middle-aged and elderly men more than women, bone turnover occurs too fast. Because of the increased activity, the affected bones feel warm through the skin and they grow bigger and clumsily shaped. Bones most likely to be involved include the shin and thigh bones, the pelvis, and the skull (where pressure by the enlarged bone on the hearing nerve can cause hearing loss). In the United States, about 1 percent of people over age forty have Paget's disease, which rarely occurs in people under age forty. The disorder is even more common in England.

> Alice had a headache—a deep ache right in the bones of her forehead. She had a pain in her left shin as well. She was sixty-six. Her doctor told her she had Paget's disease, osteitis deformans, but there was nothing to worry about. Alice was not satisfied. It hurt, but the ordinary painkillers like aspirin, Tylenol, or anti-inflammatories had no effect. The most effective way of stopping the pain of Paget's disease is with an injection of calcitonin, the other hormone made by the thyroid.

TOO MUCH CALCIUM IN THE BLOOD (HYPERCALCEMIA)

Calcitonin injections are also useful in treating hypercalcemia. This disorder may develop in Graves' disease because of the body's disturbed metabolism, in anyone bedbound for months, with the prolonged use of certain water tablets (thiazide diuretics), or as a result of excess vitamin D prescribed for medical reasons. Very occasionally someone with an underactive thyroid may have such a sluggish metabolism that calcium fails to move readily through its normal cycle but instead builds up in the blood.

In young people too much calcium can lead to acutely painful kidney stones, but in older age groups the symptoms are very different, and vague. Affected individuals suffer from fatigue for no apparent reason, weakness, low spirits, and a sense of not feeling "up to par." Often the sufferer doesn't realize how poorly he has felt until treatment with calcitonin restores him to his normal self.

OSTEOPOROSIS

Osteoporosis is a progressive decrease in density of the bones that weakens them and makes them more vulnerable to fracture. It is increasingly common after forty, especially in women. Typically, it develops when estrogen levels are drastically cut by menopause or by surgery on the ovaries, including hysterectomy with removal of the ovaries. At the same time, calcitonin levels are reduced, which is thought to be one of the causes of the disorder. Calcitonin treatment may be useful. Hormone replacement therapy (HRT) is effective, but some people cannot take it because of breast or womb conditions, a tendency to blood clots, or high blood pressure. Others choose not to take HRT, especially in light of a study published in 2002 in the *Journal of the American Medical Association* (JAMA) that showed a higher rate of heart disease among users of a particular kind of HRT.

Calcitonin to treat osteoporosis must be given either by injection (at least three times a week for six months) or via nasal spray. Bisphosphonates, which can be taken by mouth and include such prescription drugs as etidronate (Didronel) or alendronate (Fosamax), present other options for treating osteoporosis. Reports of their effectiveness are conflicting. Alendronate in particular dominates the U.S. market for osteoporosis medications, but the side effects, which can include severe upper gastrointestinal (GI) reactions, are off-putting for some. One study reports that one in three women complained of new upper GI problems after starting treatment with Fosamax.

TOO LITTLE CALCIUM IN THE BLOOD (HYPOCALCEMIA)

The parathyroid glands are intimately close neighbors of the thyroid, but quite separate. They lie behind the thyroid gland, two on each side, and each weighs about an ounce. Their delicate blood vessels run across the back of the thyroid and can easily be damaged during an operation for a goiter or tumor.

Damage to the parathyroids, either directly or through an interruption to their blood supply, causes the calcium level in the blood to plummet in an effect known as hypocalcemia. Symptoms develop within days, including muscle cramps and spasms, tingling around the mouth, and finally, convulsions. There is intense anxiety. The effects are similar to those of hyperventilation. If the symptoms persist, a few weeks on calcium tablets will resolve the situation before the condition becomes severe.

The parathyroids are most likely to be only slightly bruised or irritated by an operation on the thyroid. In the rare circumstance of permanent parathyroid hormone deficiency, calcitriol capsules, containing a synthetic vitamin-D preparation, are required. In such a case, the calcium level in the blood must be checked regularly.

Apart from parathyroid damage, hypocalcemia can result from the following:

- long-term use of estrogen-containing HRT or the contraceptive pill

- diuretics such as furosemide, which may wash too much calcium out in the urine

* some kidney problems

* anticonvulsant medicines, and some tranquillizers

* dietary problems—either not enough calcium (available from dairy foods) or an excess of whole wheat and other grains that hinder the absorption of calcium

10

Keeping Your Thyroid Happy

Your thyroid is an obliging organ. You can anticipate a lifetime of trouble-free service at minimal cost to you. It will organize the intricate workings of your whole body to fit changing circumstances. It will make swift adjustments in the face of illness, injury, or disaster, much as a car with an automatic transmission will respond to driving conditions without your having to do anything. The thyroid, however, runs a more complicated machine and is far more sensitive than an automobile. It will make immediate, medium-range, and long-term alterations to your metabolism according to what you eat, how much you use your muscles, your mood, your age, any stresses you are under—and even the weather.

What does this remarkable and priceless piece of equipment require to keep running? Its demands couldn't be more modest: an average Western diet and a supply of clean drinking water. The ingredients in your diet that are of special concern to the thyroid are iodine, a vital element used by no other organs, and various vitamins. These basics are discussed in this chapter, as are other factors potentially affecting thyroid health.

IODINE

A minute amount of iodine is sufficient to maintain optimal thyroid function, and an excess is harmful. The thyroid gland can store iodine to last for two or three months, but the daily requirement averages out to about 90 micrograms (mcg). Less than 50 mcg throws a strain on the thyroid. One response it makes is to switch production in favor of T_3 instead of the usual 90 percent T_4, since one molecule of T_3 requires only three-quarters as much iodine as one of T_4. In the United Kingdom the usual diet provides 100 to 150 mcg of iodine per day, and in the United States it supplies anywhere from 100 to 600 mcg. Micrograms are minute; a small carton of yogurt weighs about 125 grams—or 125,000,000 micrograms.

Sources of Iodine for Most of Us

- dairy products—56 percent (this is at a maximum in the spring and summer months, when dairy cows ingest fresh grass, which contains more iodine than their usual fodder)

- bread and cereals—16 percent

- meat and fish, especially saltwater fish and shellfish—11 percent

- sugar—11 percent

- drinks—4 percent

If you live by the ocean, you will even get some iodine from the air you breathe, but the water supply and locally grown vegetables will provide a negligible amount. There is a coastal area in Wales where the population used to be chronically short of iodine, due to the poor quality of the soil, similar to that commonly found in mountainous districts. In some countries, very small amounts of iodine are added to the salt or flour. Iodized salt is also still widely available in the United States. It is not thought to be necessary in Britain, although some people prefer to use sea salt in the home.

Unless you live in a remote area, where goiter is obviously prevalent, and all your food is produced on the spot, you won't have to worry about getting enough iodine. In some circumstances, however, you need to make extra sure of your supply; for women, these include the important life cycles of puberty, pregnancy, and menopause. This also applies to anyone after a physical illness, especially in the winter, or following a period of overactive thyroid. A prologed cold spell makes the thyroid work harder, which means it uses more of its raw materials. The safe ploy is to have two seafood meals a week. The top natural providers of iodine are sea fish such as halibut and whiting, sea crustaceans such as shrimp, and seaweeds like kelp. If you really can't stand fish, go for the dairy products—yogurt, cheese, butter, and milk.

VITAMINS

More than other organs, the thyroid requires an adequte supply of most vitamins. Again, this is especially important for the same key populations that need a little more iodine than usual, including pubescent girls, pregnant women, and women going through menopause. As with iodine, an excess of many vitamins can be as damaging as not enough. Your aim must be to obtain them safely via your food, not through synthetic concentrates.

Which Vitamins to Use and Where to Find Them

Vitamin A
Go for yellow—carrots, cheese, butter or margarine, egg yolk, fresh or dried apricots. Dark-green vegetables are also a good source. The thyroid has a special relationship with this vitamin. Without thyroid hormone the body cannot deal with vitamin A properly and the skin develops an allover yellowish tinge. This sometimes occurs in severe cases of anorexia nervosa, which causes thyroid-hormone levels to become drastically reduced.

The B Vitamins

There are several requirements in this group:

- ❧ *Thiamine.* This is found in whole wheat, dried beans and peas, nuts, and pork, but rice, white flour, and raw fish interfere with the body's ability to use it. The thyroid needs this vitamin to organize the metabolism of carbohydrates, our staple nutrient

- ❧ *Riboflavin.* This is found in liver, cheese, and eggs, as well as in meat and yeast extracts

- ❧ *Niacin.* This is found in liver, kidneys, eggs, yeast extract, and instant coffee

- ❧ *Vitamin B-12.* This is found in meat, poultry, liver, eggs, and milk. Beware of running low on B-12 if you are a vegetarian, and especially if there is any autoimmune illness in the family. The resulting pernicious anemia is frequently found in sufferers of Hashimoto's and Graves' diseases

- ❧ *Vitamin B-6.* This is available in almost all foods. The biggest danger is accidentally overdosing with vitamin pills

Vitamin C

Citrus fruits, peppers, lettuces, green vegetables, some berries, and some melons are all good sources of vitamin C. You need it in particular to pep up your immune system—which is all the more vital if you have been epxosed to any form of stress.

Vitamin D

Herrings, sardines, margarine, and eggs provide vitamin D, as does a regular dose of sunshine. If you are dark-skinned, you need more sun than a fair-skinned blond does to manufacture the vitamin in your skin. Unless you are specifically advised to by your doctor, don't supplement with fish-liver oils or pills—too much vitamin D is definitely dangerous.

Vitamin E

Vitamin E is found in margarine, sunflower-seed oil and other polyunsaturates, and wheat germ. No one runs short of this vitamin unless they are actually starving.

CLEAN WATER

The only other basic requirement for keeping your thyroid happy is clean, uncontaminated drinking water—something most of us can take for granted. Localized outbreaks of goiter and thyroid failure have occurred in various parts of Europe from time to time. They have been traced to pollution of water with sewage and confined to those sharing the same water supply. Michelangelo may have been right to blame his goiter on the "stagnant streams" near the Sistine Chapel.

DIETS THAT UPSET THE THYROID

Chronic Overeating

A brief binge, espeically of the sweet-tooth variety, triggers the thyroid into releasing extra T_3. This speeds up the metabolism for an hour or so, which works toward using up the excess. In response to continued overeating, however, the thyroid continues producing more T_3. The increased rate of metabolism throws a strain on the heart, circulatory system, and breathing apparatus. You know that you are overstepping the mark if your heart starts hammering and you are uncomfortably hot and slightly short of breath.

The rev-up happens only while you are still overloading your body with nourishment; it is not affected by your actual weight. You might weigh 275 pounds, but if you are eating an average diet and maintaining a stable weight, your thyroid won't react at all; your metabolic rate will be normal.

Undernutrition

While overeating puts a mild strain on the thyroid, eating too little really upsets it. If you start on a weight-loss diet or for some other reason suddenly cut down drastically on food intake, within a day or two the thyroid responds. It starts converting T_4 into inactive reverse-T_3 instead of the active hormone. The effect is an immediate reduction in the rate at which the body burns up its nourishment.

You are likely to feel cold, and because of the effect on your heart rate and circulation, you may develop a headache. You may have noticed this at the beginning of dieting or if you miss several meals consecutively for other reasons. As little as 1½ ounces of cookie, bread, or a banana will put you right straightaway. If you continue on a restricted diet, your body resets to a lower basic metabolic rate, to allow it to run economically on whatever nourishment is available.

It is T_3 that actually controls the metabolism, using T_4 that has been converted. Initially, while T_3 levels are down, your T_4 output stays near normal for some time. Eventually, if there is still a food shortage, T_4 output is reduced too. The mental and physical slowdown caused by an underactive thyroid then comes into effect.

The key to recovery is a carbohydrate diet. A meal of eight hundred calories—say pizza and apple pie—gives you a start toward normal thyroid function. A fatty diet may fill you up but does nothing to restore normality to your metabolism. A high-protein diet is only slightly better than one that is high in fat, probably because the body can make sugar out of protein, though not from fat.

It was pasta that put Stephanie back on track. She had been anxious about her finals, plus her boyfriend had broken up with her. From then on she practically lived on black coffee. Anyway, she didn't have an appetite. Instead of being on the ball, she felt dopey and couldn't concentrate on all the studying she knew she must do. Stephanie's friend Bernie saved the day by looking in on her and bringing along a pasta dish he'd made, with a Danish pastry for dessert.

The spell was broken. Stephanie felt less lethargic and depressed, and she even became hungry again for the normal diet of a student on scholarship—one with plenty of carbohydrate filler. She managed to scrape through her exams.

Too Much Iodine

Getting an excess of iodine is a rarity if you follow an ordinary diet. Exceptions have arisen from eating hamburger made from the neck of the animal, which probably included some thyroid gland by accident. After several outbreaks of thyroid and iodine-excess symptoms in the American Midwest, neck meat is no longer used for ground-beef products. In Hokkaido, Japan, where the population was in the habit of eating a seaweed called *kombu*, overdosage of iodine led to goiters and a decrease of thyroid-hormone production.

Although there may be a brief burst of thyroid overactivitiy, the usual outcome of iodine excess is to suppress the thyroid. Cows fed on sea-kale have concentrated levels of iodine in their milk, and consuming this milk has caused thyroid upsets in children. The use of iodized disinfectants in dairy work has also caused problems.

For all intents and purposes there is a negligible chance of taking in too much iodine through ordinary food in the West. Special dieter's meals and drinks, however, often contain excessive amounts of iodine, which could cause trouble if a person used them too enthusiastically. Natural-food shops sell kelp, a seaweed rich in iodine, as well as multivitamin/multimineral preparations that can poison the thyroids of health-food lovers.

An iodine-reducing diet, sometimes needed before a whole-body scan to diagnose suspected cancer, or before treatment for thyroid cancer, involves avoiding the following:

- iodized salt or sea salt

- milk and dairy products

- eggs

- seafood

- kelp tablets and other kelp-containing foods and supplements

- red food dyes (erythrosine)

Foods That Prevent the Thyroid from Using Available Iodine

Certain foods contain substances called *goitrogens*, so named because eating them in excess leads to goiter and the symptoms of underactive thyroid. They are all plant foods, and they include the following:

- cabbage and many other members of the brassica family—including brussels sprouts, cauliflower, kohlrabi, horseradish

- peanuts, walnuts, almonds

- rapeseed and mustard seed

- sweet corn, millet, sorghum

- soy—especially as part of a high-fiber diet, since the combination causes too much thyroid hormone and iodine to be excreted from the body

- cassava—a starch food that is a staple in many poorer countries

➤ milk from dairy cows that have been fed kale, rutabagas, and turnips, as has occurred in the United Kingdom

These plants contain cyanide derivatives that prevent the thyroid from taking in enough iodine. Matters are made worse if the individual uses a lot of salt. The thyroid swells as it struggles to do its work.

The only people likely to run into trouble with goitrogens are the vulnerable groups—those with a family history of thyroid disorder, pregnant women, pubertal girls, babies and young children, and the elderly—children who have less variety in their diet than most Western children do, and health enthusiasts. Moderation is the safe watchword, and risks arise in someone who indulges a craze for nuts and soy instead of more commonplace sources of protein. The goitrogens have done us a good turn, however; the original anithyroid drugs, so useful in treating Graves' disease, were developed through these plants.

MEDICINES THAT CAN CAUSE PROBLEMS

Medicines That Can Strain the Thyroid

Any of the following can interfere with the smooth workings of the gland, or at least can upset thyroid-test results:

➤ tolbutamide (Orinase), for diabetes

➤ chlorpropamide (Diabinese), also for diabetes

➤ phenylbutazone (Butacote), for ankylosing spondylitis

➤ diazepam (Valium), for anxiety

➤ heparin, to prevent clotting in heart problems

➤ lithium (Lithane, Lithonate), to prevent relapse in psychiatric illness. More than a third of people taking lithium develop underactive thyroid

- beta-blockers (Inderal), for high blood pressure

- salicylates, including aspirin (Bayer), a painkiller

- steroids (e.g., prednisolone), for any severe physical reaction

- phenothiazines (Thorazine), as an antipsychotic or tranquillizer

- amiloride (Midamor), a diuretic

- androgens (testosterone), the male sex hormone

- tamoxifen (Nolvadex), an anti-estrogen to ward off breast cancer

- sulfonamides, antibacterial drugs

- acetazolamide (Diamox), for glaucoma and fluid retention

- resorcinol, used for acne and dandruff

- para-aminosalicylic acid (PAS), for tuberculosis

All of these medicines suppress thyroid activity, lowering the level of T_4 in the blood, even if the gland is perfectly healthy. Sometimes, particularly with lithium, long-term hypothyroidism of the Hashimoto's type develops.

The following medicines have a different effect:

- phenytoin (Dilantin) and related medicines used to control epilepsy; these anticonvulsants use up the thyroid hormones unusually quickly, which may cause a shortage

- carbamazepine (Tegretol), used as an anticonvulsant, it inhibits the release of T_4 into the blood

- co-trimoxazole (Septra), used for urinary infections; it inhibits the release of T_4 into the blood

- levodopa (Dopar) and bromocriptine (Parlodel), both used for Parkinson's disease; they stop the stimulating action of TSH, leading to a shortage of T_4 and T_3

Medicines That Seem to Increase T_4 and T_3

Although neither of the following actually stimulates the production of more thyroid hormone, they seem to do so:

- estrogen (in the contraceptive pill and in HRT); it provides more of the transport protein

- furosemide-type diuretics (e.g., Lasix), by ridding the body of fluid, make the blood more concentrated so there is more thyroid hormone per milliliter

Medicines Containing Iodine

Be wary of these if you've ever had a thyroid problem, and investigate whether it could be your thyroid if you get some puzzling symptoms when you are taking one of them. These medicines are liable to give your thyroid more iodine than it can cope with. It may react at first by going into overdrive and producing too much hormone, resulting in anxiety and palipitations. The usual end result, however, is a near-complete cessation of thyroid activity, resulting in a general slowing down of the body's functions.

Amiodarone (Cordarone). This is an excellent medicine for dealing with tricky faults in the rhythm of the heart, but it causes thyroid problems in 6 percent of people taking it. These problems may be due to either underactivity or overactivity, resulting in totally different symptoms: the body's slowing to a snail's pace or racing with edgy speed. Since it takes a long time to clear amiodarone from the circulation, and since the drug may be vital for normal heart functioning, it is usually best to continue taking it, but help the thyroid by adding other drugs—for example, thyroxine in the case of underactivity, or an antithyroid such as carbimazole in the case of overactivity.

Some cough medicines. Many prescription and over-the-counter preparations contain iodine.

X-ray contrast media. Media given, for instance, for gall-bladder investigations usually contain iodine.

Povidone skin antiseptic (betadine) and tincture of iodine. Very little iodine is likely to get into the system from these, but they should be avoided during pregnancy.

Multivitamin/multimineral supplements.

YOUR GENES

Of course you cannot choose your parents or the genes they donate to you, even to make your thyroid happy. It is useful, however, to know what illnesses your family members have had. The closer the relationship, the more relevant the medical history. Any kind of thyroid disorder is important to know about, especially since the major forms—Graves' and Hashimoto's—are caused by an autoimmune reaction. Other autoimmune disorders indicate a tendency to react to stress by making antibodies against the body's own tissues, including the thyroid. Autoimmune conditions to be aware of in your family's medical history include the following:

* vitiligo—a patchy loss of pigment in the skin

* type-I diabetes—also known as insulin-dependent diabetes

* rheumatoid arthritis

❦ pernicious anemia

❦ myasthenia gravis—a rare muscle weakness

❦ lupus

❦ Parkinson's disease

Even if one of these problems is present in your family, you are by no means sure to develop it or a thyroid disorder. Awareness of your family's medical history, however, serves as a useful reminder to give your thyroid consideration and to be alert for symptoms, especially the vague ones, that could indicate that the gland is in for difficulties. As we've seen, effective treatment exists for most thyroid problems. The important thing is to recognize the possibility of a thyroid disorder and to get a checkup, especially if you are on any of the medicines or have a partiality for any of the foods known to upset the thyroid.

STRESS

The best advice here is to avoid stress as much as you can. The term *stress* can refer to a range of different situations. What they have in common is that something must give—mind or body. The effect may be mild and short-lived or may develop into a definite illness.

Stresses That Can Affect the Thyroid

Certain types of stressful situations can affect the thyroid by triggering what is known as the *stress syndrome* (see the next page). Prominent stresses that affect the thyroid include the following:

❦ starvation, including undernutrition from anorexia nervosa or drastic weight loss

❦ involvement in a traffic accident or other serious trauma

- surgery

- severe burns

- radiation, for treatment or by accident

- emotional upset, such as bereavement

- important exams

- major psychiatric illness, such as schizophrenia, mania, or severe depression—but not including Alzheimer's disease, psychopathy, or neurotic problems

- great restriction of freedom, including imprisonment

- withdrawal from heroin or alcohol

- taking amphetamines or Ecstasy

- physical illness—you can expect the thyroid to bounce back to normal as soon as your body does, except when the liver or kidneys are involved

All these stresses can rock the thyroid, calling forth at first an extra release of thyroxine, both free and the less immediately available form attached to its carrier protein. This is called the stress syndrome. It can trigger Graves' disease, but probably only if you already have the relevant antibodies in your blood, in which case the disorder most likely would have emerged at some time anyway. The boost effect of stress may be followed by a downturn in thyroid activity. For example, during an operation the levels of T_4 and T_3 shoot up, but afterwards they temporarily slip below normal.

Humans produce two specific stress hormones: adrenaline and cortisol. Adrenaline is the first-line response, and it stimulates the thyroid as well as pepping you up in general. Ongoing stress leads to the production of high levels of cortisol, the body's own steroid. Like steroid medicines, cortisol suppresses thyroid activity, and in anyone already vulnerable, the underactivity might persist. In most cases the thyroid helps you through the stress and then returns to normal.

A whole group of stressful circumstances arise in the various physical illnesses. They affect the thyroid in slightly different ways. Examples include the following:

Feverish Illness

Any illness that raises the body temperature will make the thyroid produce inactive reverse-T_3 instead of the effective hormone. This slows down the rate at which you burn up your food, which is helpful when you are already too hot and don't feel like eating much.

Common Illnesses

Everyday ailments such as cystitis (bladder infection), bronchitis, an upset stomach, and flu all lead to the low-T_3 syndrome. Less T_4 is changed into active T_3. This mechanism is in place to conserve your energy, and does not indicate any fault in the thyroid. If you notice undue lethargy and inability to concentrate lingering after the flu or some other viral illness, there is the faintest chance that Hashimoto's thyroiditis is starting up. However, it is much more likely to be the tail end of your body's and your thyroid's reaction to the infection. Tests would confirm this.

Serious Illness

Serious illness, either acute or long term—such as pneumonia, a coronary heart attack, cancer (especially of the lung), severe anorexia nervosa, diabetes, or alcoholism—all cause a reduction in both of the thyroid hormones. You may get some of the symptoms of underactive thyroid. You may look pale, feel cold and listless, and slow down mentally.

HIV

The infection alone causes no reaction in the thyroid, but in ARC-AIDS-related complex, comprising fatigue, enlarged glands, and diarrhea, T_4 is increased but T_3 reduced. The net effect is a slightly lower metabolic rate, in addition to an overall lack of vitality. In full-blown AIDS, when the illness has tightened its grip, levels of both hormones are down and no part of the body is working properly.

Abuse of Heroin, Methadone, or Other Narcotics
Depending on its severity, narcotic abuse has the effect, similar to underactive thyroid, of the body's slowly grinding to a halt all over. This reaction, caused by the thyroid, reduces the demands on the heart and other parts of the body, which is generally helpful during a bad illness. There is no point in trying to correct the lack of thyroid-hormone production; what needs treating is the underlying addiction.

In the above conditions, thyroid function reverts to normal when the physical illness improves sufficiently. That's not the case, however, with the following conditions:

Chronic Diarrhea
No matter the cause, long-term diarrhea depletes the body of thyroid hormones faster than the gland can replace them. This is a forced shortage of thyroid hormone, not a reaction to illness, and it is reasonable to use thyroxine tablets while the bowel trouble is sorted out.

Liver Disorders
Some types of inflammation of the liver—such as hepatitis—cause a brief increase of T_4 in circulation. The liver manufactures the protein that transports T_4 in the blood, and when it is irritated it may release more of this protein than usual. As a result patients may feel unexpectedly restless during the illness, but it is a temporary effect. Serious liver problems, such as alcoholic cirrhosis, put the thyroid so far out of action that, while there is a shortage of T_4, there may be no T_3 at all, according to the bood tests. In this exceptional situation it is a good idea to help out the thyroid temporarily by taking thyroxine tablets.

Autoimmune liver disorder quite often goes hand-in-hand with Hashimoto's disease, which receives treatment with thyroxine.

Kidney Disorders

Disorders of the kidney seriously interfere with the conversion of T_4 to T_3, possibly resulting in availability of less than half the usual amount of the active hormone. This shortage adds to the feelings of weakness and depression common in kidney disease. Dialysis doesn't alter the thyroid's reaction to kidney failure, but a kidney transplant restores the thyroid to normal, along with everything else.

THYROID ILLNESS ON TOP OF PHYSICAL ILLNESS

Some physical ailments are notably aggravated by a thyroid that acts up. If you have a goiter that has given you no trouble over the years, if you have had a thyroid problem in the past, or if there are autoimmune disorders in your family, do not be surprised if your doctor wants to check your thyroid if you are slow to respond to treatment for any of the illnesses reviewed below. Thyroid treatment in such cases can be life-saving, or at least life-enhancing.

High Blood Pressure

Hypertension is made worse by either an underactive or an overactive thyroid. In the former the blood vessesl may get clogged with cholesterol, necessitating increased blood pressure. In the latter the rapid heart rate directly raises the blood pressure. Either way, it is vital to make sure that the thyroid problem is recognized and fully treated.

> Madge had always been solid, in every sense of the word. She was the backbone of the local political-party headquarters, the leading light in the dramatic society, and the driving force behind her church's women's guild, the local grange, and the

summer festival. Whatever the event, Madge was at the center of it, organizing and commanding. At fifty she seemed
unstoppable. So it was odd when Madge began missing meet-
ings and then actually resigned from the secretaryship of the
residents' association.

It seemed that everything was explained when her doctor
found she had high blood pressure. No wonder she had felt
tired, said everyone. But Madge was no better after several
weeks of treatment, either in her spirits or in her blood pressure. What surprised and alerted the doctor was when Madge
came in muffled up in a wool sweater on a sunny summer day.
Thyroxine for her underactive thyroid plus a beta-blocker for
her blood pressure has restored Madge to her accustomed
dynamic self.

Coronary Heart Disease

As with hypertension, either clogged arteries from an underactive thyroid or a pressurized heart rate from an overactive thyroid urgently adds to the risks associated with coronary heart
disease. Treatment of the thyroid disorder takes top priority.

High Cholesterol and/or Triglycerides (Hyperlipidemia)

Underactive thyroid, by increasing the levels of cholesterol in the
blood, adds to the danger of this condition, which carries a possibility of stroke.

Obstructive Airways Problems

In chronic bronchitis, emphysema, and asthma, the breathing
problems are made worse by an overactive thyroid. In these cases
patients cannot take a beta-blocker to slow down the heart and
breathing rates, but an antithyroid like carbimazole, together
with the patient's usual chest treatment, will make the breathing easier and more comfortable.

Diabetes

This illness is especially difficult to control if the thyroid is overactive, so both autoimmune disorders equally deserve full treatment.

Connections Between Thyroid Disorders and Other Illnesses

Hashimoto's Disease

Hashimoto's is more common in children and others suffering from certain genetic disorders, including cystic fibrosis, Down's syndrome, Turner's syndrome, and Klinefelter's syndrome. The thyroid problem responds well to T_4 treatment in these conditions, but unfortunately T_4 treatment does not help the genetic problem.

Graves' Disorder

Graves' disorder is frequently associated with ulcerative colitis, celiac disease, Crohn's disease, and myasthenia gravis.

A NOTE FOR DIETERS: HOW TO PLAY IT RIGHT

The less reputable weight-loss clinics often dish out "magic pills" that contain a purgative, a diuretic, an appetite suppressant, and thyroxine. The first two cause a person to lose fluid (and weight) temporarily but have no effect on body fat. The thyroxine is no help either. A moderate dose has nil effect; the body's own thyroid gland stops making its hormone if adequate supplies are coming in from outside. A larger dose can put a strain on the heart and cause high blood pressure, made worse in conjunction with an appetite suppressant.

Appetite suppressants all act like amphetamines, raising the blood pressure and increasing tension as inevitable side effects. With a substantial dose of thyroxine the result can be disastrous, triggering Graves' disease, a coronary, or a nervous breakdown. It is this combined effect of drugs that accounts for the deaths, from time to time, of dieters who have fallen into the hands of the unscrupulous.

The way to make the most of your dieting efforts and of your thyroid is by employing a gentler approach. If you starve yourself—or nearly—your thyroid will work against you by immediately turning your metabolic rate down, so that you use up your food and your fat at a slower rate. It will also slow down your digestion, so that you obtain every last calorie from whatever you've eaten. In addition your body will slow down generally, so that even during exercise you will burn up fuel slowly.

It is better to reduce your weight by one to two pounds weekly as a maximum, so that the thyroid is not stimulated into adjusting your metabolic rate downwards. The thyroid does not respond to your actual weight, however unacceptable it may be to you, but rather to any sharp change in food intake. Since every meal you eat gives your thyroid a brief boost, in addition to causing an increase in metabolic rate, don't miss any meals—just change them. Cut out the fats as far as possible; don't increase the protein (meat, etc.); and don't ditch bread, potatoes, pasta, and rice—these foods provide the carbohydrates that your thyroid runs on and that keeps your metabolic rate revved up.

Chapter

11

Tests and Treatments

This chapter provides an overview of the various laboratory tests and medical treatments used in diagnosing and correcting thyroid disorders. Although many of these procedures and remedies are touched on in greater or lesser detail in earlier chapters, the summary given here is meant to serve as a convenient and ready reference tool.

Laboratory tests are particularly useful when the thyroid is misbehaving. How you feel and what you notice wrong or unusual remain the most important aspects of determining thyroid health, but they can be deceptive. Take Graves' disease: In one person it causes a goiter, loss of weight, and an anxiety state; in another, all the symptoms point to a heart disorder. A test will identify the true cause.

Reasons for having tests include the following:

* to determine if the thyroid is working normally

* to pinpoint the problem, if any

* to indicate whether the problem is mild or serious

* to help select the dosage of any medication

* to monitor progress

No test is 100 percent accurate every time, but at 95 percent accuracy, thyroid tests come close.

STANDARD THYROID TESTS

Standard thyroid tests are made on a small sample of blood, and they measure the concentration of various substances in it, including the following:

T_4—thyroxine, the main thyroid hormone. Each molecule contains four iodine atoms

T_3—triiodothyronine, the more active thyroid hormone, formed by the removal of one iodine atom from each thyroxine molecule

rT_3—reverse-T_3, an inactive type of T_3, with a different arrangment of its three iodine atoms

TSH—thyroid-stimulating hormone. This substance is made in the pituitary gland and directs the thyroid to produce its hormones. The amount of TSH goes up when the thyroid isn't providing enough T_4 and T_3 for the body's needs, and down when there is a surplus

TRH—thyroid-releasing hormone. This comes from the hypothalamus—the part of the brain that organizes sex, eating, drinking, sleeping, and the metabolism, with an input from what's happening around you and from your personal feelings and desires—and stimulates the pituitary gland to produce TSH. TRH was discovered in 1968

TBG—thyroid-binding globulin, one of the carrier proteins that act as transporters for 99.9 percent of the thyroxine in the circulation

FT_4—free thyroxine, the tiny but signficant part of T_4 hormone in the blood that is not bound up with a protein but is immediately available. The level of FT_4 is useful in assessing whether the thyroid itself is functioning properly, regardless of the amount of carrier protein

FT_3—free T_3. The test for FT_3 is available in only a few laboratories

SCREENING TESTS

Thyroid screens are administered "just in case" on all newborn babies in the West; on individuals at a key point in life, for example during pregnancy; and on anyone with symptoms that could be caused by a thyroid problem. Additionally, preventive screening in women age fifty-plus—and earlier in the at-risk groups (see the section "Subclinical Hypothyroidism," in Chapter 3, for a list of these)—can protect them from thyroid disorders. Men can wait until age sixty, if they are in good health, before undergoing regular screening tests.

The most commonly used screening tests are for T_4 and TSH, but there are several others.

T_4 Test

This measures the amount of thyroxine in the blood, both free and attached to proteins. If the reading is below 64 international units (5 standard units), it suggests an underactive thyroid; if it is more than 142 international units (11 standard units), this should mean an overactive thyroid—other things being equal. The trouble is that other things may not be equal. If there is a shortage of carrier protein, the result will be low; an excess of carrier protein will yield a higher result. Yet the thyroid may be working perfectly.

Increased protein and hence a *high* reading may be caused by the following:

- ☙ pregnancy, HRT, or the contraceptive pill (because of the extra estrogen in the system)

- ❧ hepatitis (inflammation of the liver)

- ❧ porphyria (a group of rare disorders that can affect the skin)

- ❧ cannabis

- ❧ a hereditary quirk

Reduced protein and hence a *low* reading may be caused by the following:

- ❧ steroids used to treat illness

- ❧ body-building steroids (taken by athletes)

- ❧ nephrosis (a kidney problem)

- ❧ cirrhosis of the liver

- ❧ a hereditary quirk

To determine whether an abnormally high or low T_4 level is in fact due to the thyroid, two choices exist: the TSH test or the FT_4 test.

TSH Test

The TSH test is often used instead of, rather than in addition to, the T_4 test; it is simpler for the lab than the FT_4 test. If the thyroid is failing to supply enough hormone for the body's requirements, TSH, the thyroid stimulator, comes into action to make the thyroid increase production. If the TSH result is above the critical level (2.0 or more m-IU/L, or milli–international units per liter) the thyroid simply isn't coming up with the goods; it is underactive.

On the other hand, if there is too much thyroxine, the thyroid needs little or no stimulation and the TSH level may be undetectable.

FT$_4$ Test

The FT$_4$ test is becoming increasingly popular as a true measure of thyroid activity.

TBG Test

The TBG test is seldom used, since thyroid function is adequately assessed without it.

T$_3$, FT$_3$, and R-T$_3$ Tests

A raised T$_3$ or FT$_3$ level occurs in T$_3$ toxicosis. The disorder causes the same symptoms as Graves' diseases but doesn't result in an excess of thyroxine, which is puzzling until T$_3$ levels are investigated.

Even with a healthy thyroid, increasing age causes a slow reduction in T$_3$, unlike T$_4$. A number of illnesses also have the same effect—the low-T$_3$ syndrome. Fasting, starvation, and anorexia nervosa all induce a low T$_3$ level with a corresponding increase in reverse-T$_3$.

TRH Test

Unlike the tests discussed so far, this one involves more than taking a single blood sample. It tests the pituitary gland, which programs the thyroid. Occasionally, a low T$_4$ output is caused by the pituitary's failing to secrete TSH to stimulate the thyroid. This test essentially consists of giving the patient an injection of TRH, which should stimulate a healthy pituitary to produce more TSH. The test is time-consuming but not unpleasant.

Patients are instructed to skip breakfast, then are given a preliminary blood test to determine TSH level. When the patient is lying down and mentally relaxed, she is given a TRH injection. Two odd things happen: She gets a funny taste in her mouth and a peculiar feeling low in the pelvic region, something like wanting to pass urine. Next, she is again tested for TSH after twenty, forty, and sixty minutes. Normally, the TSH level increases twenty to thirty minutes after the TRH injection and returns to its original level after sixty to ninety minutes.

If the individual has an overactive thyroid, the TSH level will fail to increase in response to the TRH injection. It may also fail to increase in people who have a pituitary disorder or in some perfectly healthy elderly men or in people undergoing serious depressive illnesses. The TRH test is therefore sometimes used in psychiatry to help with a diagnosis of depression, but an ordinary TSH test is simpler and just as useful to detect thyroid problems.

Antibody Tests

From the patient's perspective, these are simple—ordinary blood tests. For the laboratory, they are complex. Antibodies in the blood indicate susceptibility to the following autoimmune thyroid problems:

Graves' Disease
The main antibody responsible for this condition is TRAb, thyroid receptor antibody. If a high level of this antibody is present during pregnancy, it is a serious warning to take action to protect the unborn baby.

Hashimoto's Disease
Several antibodies are involved in Hashimoto's disease, including anti-TG (antithyroglobulin) and anti-M (antimicrosomal). Ninety percent of Hashimoto's sufferers carry these antibodies, but so do one in five people who have never had a thyroid problem. Members of this last group, however, may be more susceptible to developing an autoimmune disorder if their thyroid is put under stress, for instance by lithium medication, an infection, or a faulty diet.

Radioactive Iodine Uptake (RAIU) Test

This is a test of how effectively or hungrily the thyroid cells are latching on to the iodine in circulation, which is a necessary ingredient of thyroid hormones. The test begins with a scan of the patient's basic level of radioactivitiy, using a sort of Geiger counter. Then he or she is given a measured dose of a mildly radioactive form of iodine, ^{123}I, in a capsule or as a liquid. The thyroid area is then scanned again at various intervals for up to twenty-four hours to see how much of the iodine has been taken up. For a quicker test, the follow-up scan can be done three to four hours after the start, but in this case the patient must do without food during that time.

The results are useful in diagnosis and also in assessing the dosage necessary if radioactive iodine treatment is in view.

High uptake will result from the following:

- Graves' disease and other overactivity

- iodine deficiency

- having stopped taking antithyroid drugs

- a diet full of soy

- kidney disease

Low uptake will result from the following:

- an underactive thyroid

- medicines containing iodine

- a diet high in iodine-enriched foods or vitamin/mineral products

- taking thyroxine (patients must stop taking it for one month before the test)

- previous radioactive iodine treatment or a thyroid operation

- old age

- having just exercised very energetically

The radioactive iodine used for the RAIU test has nothing like the strength used in treatment. Its radioactivity only lasts three or four days. Another radioactive material, technetium, is sometimes used instead of iodine; it is given by injection. Whichever material is used, even at this low level of radiation, the test is unsuitable for young children or anyone who might become pregnant.

Scintigram

This technique uses a special camera to produce a brightly multicolored picture showing where iodine is taken up by thyroid tissue, and how vigorously. Like the RAIU test, it depends on first being given a measured amount of the weak radioactive iodine ^{123}I or technetium 99m. In a few centers, fluorescent scanning is available; this measures ordinary, nonradioactive iodine through something like an X ray, and almost no radiation is involved.

A scintigram is useful

- to show the size and shape of the gland

- to check for thyroid tissue behind the breastbone

- to find out whether a lump in the tongue or neck is thyroid tissue that has gone off course during development

- most importantly, to provide information on a particular knob or lump of tissue in the thyroid, with possible results as follows:

  - a "hot" nodule (showing as red) is overactive, taking in a lot of iodine

  - a "warm" nodule (showing as orange-yellow) is normally active

  - a "cold" nodule (showing as greenish) is not taking up iodine and may be a cyst or a tumor. This calls for further investigation to exclude cancer.

X Ray

An ordinary X ray gives a shadowy image of the size and position of the thyroid. In particular, a chest X ray may reveal a shadow behind the breastbone that could be an extension of thyroid tissue. Ultrasound, a CT scan, or a scintigram will be needed for more precise information.

Barium Swallow

This is an X ray taken while the patient swallows a barium drink that shows up on X ray. It reveals any pressure on the gullet.

CT (Computerized Tomography) Scan

This is an X ray that presents a cross-sectional image of the neck or other area of the body.

Ultrasound

This is a simple, painless method of obtaining a picture of an internal organ, including the thyroid. It is perfectly safe for pregnant mothers or children. It produces a moving picture by processing the echo of a high-frequency sound—too high for the human ear—projected onto the organ. The echoes vary depending on the consistency of the tissues under the skin. The principle involved is something like that behind distinguishing between a piece of wood, a tin can, and a cushion by tapping them. A normal thyroid is solid but not hard, and is unlike a cyst full of fluid. The technological magic lies in converting the inaudible echoes into visible pictures.

The procedure is pleasant enough. The patient lies down, and her neck is anointed with a lubricating gel or oil. The sensitive endpiece of the apparatus then easily slides over the skin, and that's all the patient feels.

In addition to distinguishing a cyst from solid tissue, the ultrasound provides a moving image of the organs and structures in the neck. This information is invaluable for guiding the needle when a biopsy of a particular part of the thyroid is required.

Fine-Needle Aspiration (FNA)

FNA is a neat method of doing a biopsy—that is, obtaining a sample of tissue to examine under the microscope and identify precisely. It is safe, simple, and quick. The patient lies down with a small pillow under the shoulders. A local anesthetic may be used, but the aspiration by itself is almost painless. A fine needle with a syringe attached is slipped into the part of the thyroid (or other body part) to be investigated, and a tiny sample of tissue is withdrawn.

If it is a very small nodule that is to be examined, an ultrasound will allow the operator to see exactly where the tip of the needle is positioned throughout the procedure.

The great value of FNA is for distinguishing between a commonplace nodule of normal thyroid tissue, a harmless cyst or benign growth, and a cancer. This knowledge is a signpost to the best form of treatment.

Metabolic Rate

Although the main work of the thyroid is controlling the rate at which the bodily processes use up the available nourishment, the metabolic rate is seldom tested. Up until now there has been no quick and simple method for doing so, but technology is catching up.

A metabolic test is useful in research studies. Its purpose is to assess the amount of oxygen an individual uses minute by mintue. Oxygen use increases immediately after a meal. You may notice that you feel warmer just after eating, even if you ate cold food; this is because of the increased degree of slow combustion going on inside of you.

A raised BMR (basic metabolic rate) goes with overactivity of the thyroid and accounts for the person who eats enormously and stays thin. The opposite happens with an underactive thyroid.

Electrocardiogram

This electrical tracing of the heart's activity is the standard method of assessing how well the heart is working. It shows characteristic changes in overactive and underactive thyroid.

Ophthalmic Curve Meter

This apparatus measures the degree of protrusion of the eye or eyes and is useful for confirming a diagnosis of hyperthyroidism.

TREATMENT FOR AN UNDERACTIVE THYROID

The aim in treating underactive thyroid, or hypothyroidism, is to restore normal levels of thyroid hormone as soon as possible. If you are a young, healthy adult and haven't been ill for more than a few months, you can start with a reasonably large dose of synthetic thyroxine—say 100 micrograms (mcg) daily, encased in one tiny white tablet. Usually this will need to be adjusted upward after the first month or two. Subsequently, the doctor will allow longer intervals between checkups and blood tests.

Special Circumstances

Some patients require special consideration when determining dosage. Half doses for the first month are given to

- those with years-long thyroid-hormone shortages

- those over forty-five and healthy

  Quarter doses for the first month are given to

- those over forty and with severe thyroid-hormone shortages

❧ those with heart problems

Other special cases include

❧ following radioactive iodine treatment or surgery, when it takes several weeks for the remaining thyroid to settle and for the dosage of T_4 to be worked out

❧ patients age seventy-plus, for whom smaller doses are adequate

❧ babies, who need full dosage (based on their size) from day one

❧ children up to five years old, who need relatively high doses

Subclinical Hypothyroidism

Patients with subclinical hypothyroidism feel perfectly well, but a routine screening reveals that they have high TSH, indicating some thyroid hormone shortage. Their doctor may give them a trial course of thyroxine or may prefer just to keep an eye on their progress.

> This is what happened with Vivienne. A high TSH reading per- sisted for over a year after she had her last baby, but it wasn't until she was in her forties, ten years later, and had just suf- fered a bout of gastroenteritis that the symptoms of hypothy- roidism appeared.

How Long to Continue with the Treatment

Medication for an underactive thyroid is usually required for life. The dose that keeps a person feeling well and keeps her TSH level normal should be continued, with a checkup and blood test every six to twelve months. It may be possible to reduce the dose as she grows older.

Effects, Good and Bad

Although the effects of thyroxine begin within hours of taking the first tablet, patients will not notice any change for four or five days. Soon, however, she will notice the following:

- Pulse speeds up, improving circulation

- Temperature returns to normal so the person feels warmer

- Patient passes a lot of urine in the first two or three days, because the body has stored too much

- Patient feels lighter because of this fluid loss, and her weight continues to drop a little as she sheds surplus fat

- Appearance improves—the body loses its unsightly puffiness, and the face becomes more expressive. Gradually the skin becomes softer and smoother and newer-looking, and the yellowish tinge disappears

- Patient is livelier, more alert, happier

- Speech becomes faster and clearer within a week

- Appetite improves

- Patient wants to drink more fluids, because she is losing moisture through perspiration

- Bowels move more freely, and menstrual periods are no longer heavy and irregular

- The amount of cholesterol in the blood diminishes, and any anemia improves

Recovery from underactive thyroid is like the fairy-tale transformation of the frog into the handsome prince—or the beautiful princess.

Of course, taking too much thyroxine can lead to any of the symptoms of overactive thyroid. If the dosage is built up too quickly, angina pains may crop up in those already susceptible; this is a signal to reduce the dose. Pains in other muscles arise fairly frequently in the first few weeks of treatment, but these are temporary and harmless, though unpleasant. If the individual is diabetic, as her metabolism speeds up with the T_4, she may need more insulin or other medication to control her blood-sugar level. On the other hand, if she is taking digoxin for a heart condition, she may find that she requires less. The doctor will advise you about your particular case.

Myxedema Coma

This is a medical emergency, and there is no time to do tests before starting treatment. A single huge dose of thyroxine (300 to 500 mcg) by injection or through a tube to the stomach and no more thyroid hormones for a week is favored by some specialists; others prefer smaller doses of T_3, which acts more quickly, or T_4 given daily. Heart, breathing, and kidney functions may all need support, while hypothermia must be dealt with slowly and cautiously. It is only in the hospital that the facilities exist to adequately treat this serious effect of late-stage hypothyroidism.

TREATMENT FOR AN OVERACTIVE THYROID

Antithyroid Drugs

It was during the Second World War that the first drugs for controlling thyroid overactivity were discovered—the antithyroids. They prevent the formation of thyroid hormones while you are taking them, but only in a minority of people do the effects continue if the medication is stopped. The most common antithyroid medications are methimazole, propylthiouracil (PTU), and carbimazole. The last two also inhibit the conversion of T_4 into the more active T_3 and the formation of the anitithyroid antibodies responsible for Graves' disease.

Uses

Most people with overactive thyroid who are under forty-five are given a trial of an antithyroid before any other treatment is used; a quarter of them are generally cured. The others may need several courses to effect a permanent cure, or may remain on the medicine indefinitely, unless or until they decide to go for radioactive iodine therapy or surgery.

How Long to Continue with the Treatment

Antithyroids have to be taken regularly several times a day, particularly during the early weeks of treatment, since they do not last long in the body. This is especially important in severe cases. The dose can be increased if necessary. At best it takes four to six weeks to get the thyroid under some sort of control. By this stage, the patient can usually settle into a routine of taking the medicine every six to eight hours, and with PTU she may be able to remain free of symptoms on a once-daily regimen.

Usually people stay on the course for a year, but mildly affected individuals might wish to try reducing the dose after six months.

In over 60 percent of cases the symptoms creep back after three or four months, even after taking twelve months of medication. Some people go the other way and gradually slip into hypothyroidism; a sign of this happening is an increase in size of the goiter.

Effects, Good and Bad

Beneficial effects include the disappearance of anxiety, tremor, palpitations, weight loss, and the other symptoms of overactive thyroid.

Unfortunately, some people are sensitive to antithyroid drugs. The most common reactions are a slightly raised temperature and a blotchy-red, itchy rash. There may be odd pains that move from joint to joint, and swelling of the glands.

A more serious development is an interference with the production of white blood cells, an important part of the body's defense against infection. A sore throat and feeling vaguely under par are the early warning signs of this condition, which is called *agranulocytosis*. These symptoms call for an urgent visit to the doctor, a blood test, and stopping the medication. The patient can then either switch to a different antithyroid or try radioactive iodine treatment.

> Marion was eighteen. She had been diabetic since age eleven, and she went to her doctor because she found that she was needing more and more insulin. The doctor noticed that she was sweating, her pulse was rapid—over one hundred beats a minute instead of around sixty-five—and she had a small goiter. Tests showed an overactive thyroid, and Marion was put on PTU—propylthiouracil. This seemed to suit her: Her insulin needs settled back to normal and she felt more relaxed.
>
> In the autumn she went away to university. She continued with PTU but did not bother to visit the college clinic. When she saw her family doctor during summer vacation the next year, he noticed she had put on weight, looked puffy, and was complaining about constantly feeling tired—at age nineteen! Her thyroid was bigger. The medication was stopped, and a blood test showed not only a low T_4 but a dangerous reduction in white blood cells, the body's immune protectors. Marion acted surprisingly laid back about the whole affair. The doctor was relieved when Marion's blood count started improving within days of withholding the antithyroid. After a month the goiter had shrunk to half its previous size, and Marion became her normal, lively self.
>
> Now Marion is nearing the end of her schooling, and the whole thyroid saga is history. She is on no medication for her thyroid, and she shows no signs of too much or too little hormone. Nevertheless, it is clear that this young woman will be

susceptible to autoimmune disorders all her life—especially when she is under some physical or psychological strain. There is a close association between Marion's autoimmune type of diabetes (insulin-dependent) and both Graves' and Hashimoto's disorders.

Apart from their use as a control and a possible cure for over-active thyroid, antithyroids are frequently used on a short-term basis in preparation for treatment with radioactive iodine or surgery. The side effects are less likely to cause trouble during so limited a period.

Beta-Blockers

These modern drugs are commonly used for treating angina, high blood pressure, anxiety states, tremor, overactive thyroid, and sometimes migraine. They block the stimulating nerve pathways of the autonomic nervous system—the network that controls the heartbeat and other bodily functions we take for granted. The first and standard beta-blocker is propranolol; others are nadolol, atenolol, and metoprolol. They have no direct effect on the thyroid, except to mildly inhibit the conversion of T_4 to T_3, but they are useful in treating overactive thyroid because of their other benefits, such as calming the mood, slowing the pulse rate, and reducing blood pressure.

Because they act quickly, beta-blockers are helpful in the early stages of treatment in Graves' disease, before the antithyroid has taken effect, but they are not suitable for prolonged use or as the only treatment, since they have no curative value. They are often useful during the preparation period before radioactive iodine or surgical treatment, when the overactivity of the gland must be calmed down. People who are sensitive to antithyroids rely on beta-blockers for this purpose.

How to Take Them
Beta-blockers come as capsules or tablets. Some of them have to be taken several times a day, but once you have established the

dosage that suits you, you can change to slow-release formulations that need to be taken only once a day.

Precautions

You must not take beta-blockers if you are asthmatic or have ever had an obstructive airways disease or a heart blockage. They are not suitable if you are breast-feeding or in the last weeks of pregnancy, and they tend to make diabetes slightly worse. Some medicines do not mix well with beta-blockers, so remind your doctor if you are on any of the following: amiodarone, tranquilizers, sleep aids, antidiabetic drugs, or diuretics—and go easy on the alcohol.

Effects, Good and Bad

On the plus side are a restful slowing of the heart rate, calming down of palpitations or tremor, and keeping cool physically and emotionally. The side effects, which affect only a minority, include stomach disturbance, feeling drained, difficulty with erections (for men), bad dreams, and very occasionally a rash or dry eyes. These unpleasant symptoms improve as soon as you stop taking the medicine.

Iodine or Iodide

Iodine or iodide is used as the final tuning-up before either a thyroid operation for overactive thyroid or treatment with radioactive iodine. Either is given three times a day in a capsule, or more often as drops of Lugol's solution in milk or water, and for no more than ten days maximum.

Effects, Good and Bad

Each rapidly cuts the production of thyroid hormones, but loses its effect within a few weeks. People who are sensitive to it may react with a runny nose, headache, sore eyes, or a rash. It is not suitable for anyone pregnant or breast-feeding and would thoroughly upset the thyroid if a person stayed on it too long.

Radioactive Iodine

Radioactive iodine (^{131}I) has revolutionized thyroid treatment, replacing the disappointing antithyroid drugs, which nearly always fail in the end, and making unnecessary in most cases the difficult operation for removing part or all of the gland. One dose of radioactive iodine, or at most two or three, is all that is needed to tame the most unruly overactive thyroid. No overnight hospital stay is required.

Precautions

Patients who are pregnant or breast-feeding cannot undergo this treatment. In fact, for women in the reproductive age range, it is safest to have a pregnancy test first and then to take the treatment in the first ten days of their monthly cycle. Additionally, women should not plan a pregnancy for six months after receiving the treatment, and should take active precautions against pregnancy during that time frame. Apart from these circumstances, no age or sex is a barrier to getting this treatment; specifically, radioactive iodine can be given safely to growing children.

Who Should Take It?

This is the preferred treatment for Graves' disease, toxic multinodular goiter, and single-nodule goiter. It is also used in thyroid cancers as a fail-safe follow-up to surgery. It doesn't help in de Quervain's thyroiditis (see Chapter 2), and in Graves' disease with severe eye problems, it could possibly make them worse.

Preliminaries

To guard against the dangerous reaction of thyroid storm—a major upset of the gland in reaction to a sudden change in production of thyroid hormone (see Chapter 5)—patients with even a moderately severely overactive thyroid must take the edge off the disorder before they undergo treatment with radioactive iodine. For two to eight weeks before scheduled treatment, patients undergo a course of one of the antithyroid drugs, such as carbimazole. The antithyroid regimen ends three or four days before radioactive iodine treatment, to ensure that the thyroid will take in as much of the medicine as possible. Some doctors may also prescribe propranolol and, in the last ten days before the end of the course of antithyroid drugs, iodine drops.

The dosage of radioactive iodine will be worked out in advance according to the individual's size and the severity of her symptoms. Determining dosage may be assisted by a radioactive iodine uptake (RAIU) test, which would have to be administered before the antithyroid drug was started (see "Screening Tests," starting on page 169).

Taking Radioactive Iodine
Taking radioactive iodine couldn't be simpler: You swallow it in a drink or as capsules and go home the same day. You remain slightly radioactive to other people for a few days, and must take a few simple precautions for their sake (see page 72 for details).

Effects, Good and Bad
The benefits aren't instant, but there is a 50 to 70 percent chance of having a normally working thyroid gland within two months, and the goiter will have become visibly smaller. If the overactivity symptoms—weight loss, palpitations, anxiety, fast pulse, loose stool, etc.—are still with you, it is easy to have another dose of the medicine. The chances of a relapse are almost nil, compared with 10 percent after an operation and 60 percent with antithyroid medication.

You may get a feeling of warmth or discomfort in your neck temporarily after radioactive iodine, and occasionally the sudden change from too much T_4 to too little may bring on aching and stiffness in your muscles and joints. This is quickly cured by a short course of thyroxine tablets. The most likely unwanted effect of the radioactive iodine treatment is the development of underactivity of the thyroid. The symptoms may appear after a few months and recover without help over another few weeks, or they may develop over some years and remain permanently (see below).

Some people notice a thinning of their hair two to three months after treatment with radioactive iodine. This is more a part of the recovery process than a side effect. It is temporary and requires no treatment.

Follow-Up Treatment

Sometimes there is a blip of increased excess-thyroid symptoms immediately after taking radioactive iodine, but in any case the original symptoms will reappear. They are likely to take some weeks to subside, as the radioactivity takes effect. You can take a beta-blocker right away to tide you over this period, and after a couple of weeks you can take an antithyroid again, until it is no longer necessary.

If the thyroid reacts after radioactive iodine treatment by switching down almost at once into underactvity, it is not usually worthwhile to take thyroxine for what may be a short-lived reduction in hormone production. If, on the other hand, you have persistently low thyroxine with the accompanying symptoms, then you certainly need to start taking the tablets—probably for life. Fortunately, they are very little trouble to deal with.

Surgical Treatment

Surgical removal of part of the thyroid gland, performed under a general anesthetic, cuts down on overproduction of the hormones and is an effective cure for Graves' disease and the other types of overactivity. It is the obvious choice if radioactive iodine is ruled out. This may occur because of a pregnancy, either planned or underway, or because of work or study commitments that render impractical the prolonged medical follow-up necessary with radioactive iodine. Additionally, anyone with severe eye symptoms may not care to risk the possibility of having radioactive iodine make them worse. Other reasons to choose surgery are a large, unsightly, or awkwardly situated goiter or a suspicion of cancer.

Surgery is inadvisable for anyone with serious heart or chest problems, or for anyone in the last three months of pregnancy.

Preliminaries

To reduce the risk of thyroid storm (see Chapter 5), much the same precautions are needed as before radioactive iodine treatment. An antithyroid is given for some weeks—as long as it takes to settle the thyroid to near-normality—and, in the last week or ten days before the operation, iodine drops are added. With surgery there is no need to stop taking these medicines days before the operation.

Effects, Good and Bad

Surgery is the quickest way to permanently be rid of the symptoms of overactive thyroid. Nowadays it is an extremely safe operation, but a few possible complications do exist, including the following:

- *Damage to vocal cords.* The nerves to the vocal cords run across the thyroid, and may be bruised, irritated, or even cut during surgery. The effect is a husky voice, which usually recovers over a few months. Repair of a seriously damaged nerve may be made around two or three months later

- *Low calcium in the blood (hypocalcemia).* In a small minority of cases the calcium-controlling parathyroid glands are damaged by thyroid surgery. This results in a shortage of calcium circulating in the blood, resulting in symptoms including numbness around the mouth, tingling, and muscle cramps. Calcium tablets, or a calcium injection, can put matters right. Long-term lack of parathyroid hormone can also occur and calls for different management (see Chapter 9)

- *Underactive thyroid.* Some people, though not as many as with radioactive iodine treatment, gradually slip into hypothyroidism and require indefinite hormone replacement in the form of thyroxine

TREATMENT OF THYROID CANCER

An operation to remove the tumor and surrounding tissue is the first step in treating thyroid cancer, and no preliminary antithyroid treatment is needed. Afterward, high doses of radioactive iodine—double the dose used for treating Graves' disease—are given to nullify any remaining harmful thyroid cells. If for some reason surgery should be avoided, for instance a bad heart, radioactive iodine treatment alone is effective. It is also useful for locating and dealing with any secondary tumors that might appear.

Effects, Good and Bad
In most types of thyroid cancer, the cancerous tissue and some natural thyroid is removed or put out of action. The success rate tops 90 percent. The unwanted effects include temporary swelling and discomfort in the neck, and sometimes a brief surge of thyroid hormone into the bloodstream, which speeds up the heart and causes anxiety feelings. This settles within days. The other unwanted reactions that can occur soon after surgery are headache and muscle and joint problems. They are a reminder to start on thyroxine tablets, which will deal with the symptoms and which the patient will require for the indefinite future.

TREATMENT OF GOITER

If you have a goiter, the first necessity is a T_4 or TSH test to find out whether the thyroid is underactive or overactive.

Smooth, Symmetrical Enlargement

If the thyroid is underactive, the treatment is thyroxine tablets. If it's overactive, antithyroid medication or radioactive iodine treatment is called for. If the gland is functioning normally, you can ignore the situation, or you may opt for a six-month trial of T_4 to see if it will induce the goiter to shrink. Keep alert for any symptoms of too much thyroid activity—palpitations, anxiety, and tremor.

If the goiter is very large, uncomfortable, or ugly, and it fails to shrink with medical treatment, surgery is the only option.

Irregular, Knobby Goiter

If the goiter is small, it may shrink sufficiently with thyroxine in the case of an underactive or normal gland, or with antithyroid drugs or radioactive iodine if it is overactive. Most likely these treatments won't change the size and look of the goiter, so if it is troubling you at all, you should get it surgically removed and take T_4 hormone replacement if necessary.

Single Nodule

It is nearly always safest and best to have a single thyroid nodule removed, since you can never be sure whether it might become cancerous. The operation involved isn't serious, since only the nodule needs to go.

Endemic and Iodine-Deficiency Goiters

Millions of people in Asia and Africa have these goiters, and in some regions they are accepted as normal. They can become enormous, but the worst aspect is that many are associated with a devastating deficiency of thyroid hormones. Affected children are stunted and mentally impaired, and affected adults are dull and squat.

Effective treatment must be preventive, and it usually consists of the large-scale distribution of salt, bread, or some other staple that has been iodized, plus a cleaning-up of water supplies. Highly successful programs have been instituted in Switzerland, Mexico, and Argentina.

Supplemental iodine in the form of iodized oil, administered by injection and lasting three years, or by mouth and lasting three months, is useful in the preventive treatment of pregnant women and young children who live in the less developed parts of the world.

TREATMENT OF EYE PROBLEMS

Thyroid-related eye problems arise mainly in Graves' disease but occasionally in Hashimoto's disease. In either case they are caused by a special autoimmune process. Smoking has been proven to make eye problems more likely, or to worsen them if they are already present. Cutting out smoking is a must.

Mild Cases

Mild eye problems need only mild treatment, administered while the thyroid disorder itself is being brought under control. Dark glasses with flaps on the sides to protect the eyes from irritating gusts of wind and dust are helpful. Artificial tears, applied every two to three hours, keep the surface of the eye lubricated and soothed. Racing goggles, such as the ones swimmers use, look weird but may help, and the eyes may be more comfortable if the affected individual sleeps with the head of the bed raised a few inches. Some people find that the swelling reduces if they take diuretics. In any event, in mild cases the outlook is usually excellent.

Severe Cases

For severe eye problems, several lines of treatment exist. Steroids are usually given to reduce the swelling, in a regimen that tapers off over two months, but if you are over fifty you may not be able to take full doses of steroids because of side effects like raised blood pressure. Radiation therapy is effective in more than half of those for whom other treatment has failed; in fact, some physicians make radiation their first choice. Surgery creates more room for the eye by removing one or more walls of the orbit. This is called orbital depression. However, a second operation is often necessary to bring the eye muscles into balance. Of course, decreasing the level of thyroid overactivity is also important, but unfortunately it is not the whole answer for serious eye problems.

GENERAL TREATMENT FOR THYROID SUFFERERS

Although receiving the proper treatment for the specific thyroid ailment in question is vital, so also is comprehensive physical and psychological care. All the disorders that affect the thyroid are both physically and emotionally upsetting in a variety of ways. While you are struggling to recover in the early days of treatment, whether by taking tablets or by some other, more dramatic means, allow yourself to indulge in a convalescent lifestyle.

For a start, you need adequate rest, in a nonstressful surrounding. Perhaps your body has been under strain, trying to perform all its usual tasks without enough thyroid hormone for any part of it to run properly. Or if you suffered from an overactive thyroid, your body may have been functioning at breakneck speed to the point of exhaustion.

To help you achieve regular sleep at night, some of the daytime must be spent in exercise—the sort done indoors to limber up, complemented by walking or any sport you enjoy doing in the fresh air. The diet must be sufficiently varied to naturally include all the necessary vitamins and minerals (see Chapter 10 for a discussion of these), with plenty of fruits, vegetables, and protein. Fats are not particularly useful, and they are definitely to be avoided if your thyroid has not been making enough hormone. In general, if your thyroid is recovering from overactivity, you should eat more than most people would eat while you build up what you have lost. If your thyroid was underactive you don't need to alter your food intake; the increase in metabolic rate from the extra thyroxine will be enough to level out your weight.

The strain on the emotional system will tend to move you toward depression if you have had too little thyroid hormone, or toward anxiety if you have had too much. Either way, strands of both moods will be mixed together. Whichever way your thyroid has malfunctioned, your concentration, attention span, and short-term memory will be substandard. You might easily lose your temper or burst into tears, and you will lack your usual efficiency. All this adds up to real emotional suffering, and the treatment calls for a temporary lifting of day-to-day responsibilities, plus outpourings of sympathy, support, and encouragement from your loved ones and friends. Remember that it is not a forever situation, and you will get back to normal all the sooner if at this stage you avoid any temptation to take on every task or to make every decision.

If anyone offers to spoil you for a brief period, accept it. If no one else does, spoil yourself. Consider your comfort and pleasure first, postpone dealing with problems or making major plans, and concentrate on gentle diversions. Spend time with people who make you feel relaxed. You didn't choose to be ill, so for a few weeks cash in on the bonus side of a gentle, therapeutic, self-indulgent recovery.

Resources

THYROID ORGANIZATIONS

American Thyroid Association
6066 Leesburg Pike, Ste. 650
Falls Church VA 22041
(703) 998-8890
E-mail: admin@thyroid.org
Website: www.thyroid.org

The Endocrine Society
4350 East West Hwy., Ste. 500
Bethesda MD 20814-4426
(301) 941-0200
Fax: (301) 941-0259
E-mail: endostaff@endo-society.org
Website: www.endo-society.org

National Graves' Disease Foundation
PO Box 1969
Brevard NC 28712
(828) 877-5251
Fax: (828) 877-5250
E-mail: ngdf@citcom.net
Link for professional information: www.ngdf.org/medical.htm

The Thyroid Foundation of America
410 Stuart St.
Boston MA 02116
(800) 832-8321
Fax: (617) 534-1515
E-mail: info@allthyroid.org
Website: www.allthyroid.org

The Thyroid Society for Education and Research
7515 South Main St., Ste. 545
Houston TX 77030
(800) THYROID (849-7643)
(713) 799-9909
E-mail: help@the-thyroid-society.org
Website: www.the-thyroid-society.org
The society is a national nonprofit organization pursuing the prevention, treatment, and cure of thyroid disease.

ThyCa: Thyroid Cancer Survivors Association Inc.
PO Box 1545
New York NY 10159
(877) 588-7904
Fax: (503) 905-9725
E-mail: thyca@thyca.org
Website: www.thyca.org
The association is an all-volunteer, nonprofit organization dedicated to the support of thyroid cancer survivors, their families, and their friends. Its website was created and is maintained by thyroid cancer survivors and promotes a network of survivors, their families, and health-care professionals. The organization's aims are:

- To educate, leading to better understanding of the disease
- To share, helping others to learn from survivors' experience and knowledge
- To communicate, especially between health-care professionals, so as to better understand each others' needs
- To serve as a resource for anyone interested in thyroid cancer issues

Thyroid Foundation of Canada
PO Box/CP 1919 Stn Main
Kingston ON K7L 5J7
Canada
(800) 267-8822 (toll-free in Canada)
(613) 544-8364
Fax: (613) 544-9713
Website: www.thyroid.ca

Index